Natural Remedies

Quick Reference Guide

REGAIN BACK YOUR GOOD HEALTH

Katia Cherisol RN, ND

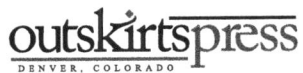
outskirtspress
DENVER, COLORADO

Natural Remedies Quick Reference Guide
Regain Back Your Good Health
All Rights Reserved.
Copyright © 2014 Katia Cherisol RN, ND
v1.0

Outskirts Press, Inc.
http://www.outskirtspress.com

ISBN: 978-1-4787-4260-9

Outskirts Press and the "OP" logo are trademarks belonging to Outskirts Press, Inc.

PRINTED IN THE UNITED STATES OF AMERICA

ACKNOWLEDGMENT

The inspiration to put this guide together was a gradual process, more like a miracle. I want to thank the one and only living God, creator of heaven and earth for the circumstances of life that inspired me to put this guide together. Eighteen years ago our family of seven found ourselves without medical insurance. In desperation my husband and I knew that we had to keep the family healthy. Being an RN I began to delve into the natural remedy books in order to treat my family on my own. It was a difficult search; I discovered that I had to dig into five to ten books for each illness. That is when I began to realize the necessity of putting a quick reference guide together for the family. I became so engross in it that I researched and began my studies as a Naturopath Doctor. In conclusion I want to thank the almighty God for his divine providential workings in our lives witch led to the publishing of this book.

DISEASE CAN BE SUCCESSFULLY TREATED AND CURED

Western society is suffering from so many diseases despite advance in modern technology. We are equipped with the finest diagnostic tools available on this planet yet the rate of disease continues to rise. Advance technology causes one to become too dependent on artificial means of disease treatment, which the human cells are unable to process. Instead of curing diseases we simply camouflage or more the symptoms to one system to another. In many cases modern way of treating disease actually adds to the distress of the system and secondary disease is formed from the actual modern treatments.

In conclusion, modern medical science needs to re-think their approach in treating disease. We have tried for decades to use modern technological laboratory techniques to disease approach. We need to realize that the human body in an incredible created machinery, capable of self-repair if given the right tools. The human body becomes diseased because it is being abused in many cases with intake of toxic material. In addition to the bombardment of toxic materials the system is suffering from nutritional deficiencies. As described in this dissertation medical science needs to be reeducated on curing diseases and not merely covering symptoms as they occur. Diseases individuals need to be educated so that they can understand the disease process and assisted in lifestyle changes which can reverse the disease process.

After working for 30 years in the secular medical field as an RN I concluded that traditional means of dealing with disease are unsuccessful. The sorrow of watching individual suffer year after years with little remedy have prompted my research for a solution. These are the incidents which prompted me to venture into a career as a Naturopath Doctor so that I can help society fight this battle on health. This book is a compilation of 15 years of research. I wanted to put a tool in the hands of those who are willing to help fight this disease battle.

CONTENTS

PREFACE

Advance Technological Effect on Dietary intake on Health

One may feel content thinking that by taking nutritional supplements they are contributing to good health not knowing they are in effect harming themselves. The fact is that vitamin supplements contain dangerous additives such as talc, dyes, sodium benzoate, methylcellulose, carnauba wax, silicon and or titanium dioxide. Vitamin supplements came in the market in the 1930's. In the 1940's however they began to make the supplements out of synthetic materials. Synthetic nutritional supplements contain aspartame which can cause irritable bowel syndrome and cancer. Research shows that synthetic vitamin D deposits toxic minerals in the heart, lungs and kidneys because it is made from coal tar derivative, irradiated cattle brain, chemical additives and formaldehyde.

Due to the overwork of soil secondary to industrial farming we are facing a crisis of soil nutrient deficiency. The use of machinery, fertilizers and other farm chemicals and plant breeding have caused a major problem with soil nutrient deficiency along with water and air pollution. Moreover chemical farming produces less nutrient food products. This soil depletion also affects the farm animals. Because the food needed to feed farm animals are depleted farmers have resorted to hormone injections and other artificial means of feed in the farm animals that are place in the market for food consumption. The consumption of these products creates nutritional deficiency and disease in humans.

Trans Fat poses a health risk. Saturated and Trans fats raises LDL (bad cholesterol), levels in the blood. These fat increases the risk of heart disease. In 1957 the American Heart Association proposes a reduction in dietary saturated fats, such as are found in beef, butter in an attempt to reduce heart disease risk. Trans fats causes and elevated blood cholesterol levels, these fats can deposit in the walls of blood vessels leading to a condition called atherosclerosis. This cell wall fat deposit causes a narrowing of the blood vessel lead to various health conditions including heart disease, heart attack and premature death. Cholesterol is only found in animal products, hence if one is concerned regarding cholesterol levels, eliminating all animal products would be a start.

There has been a growing concern regarding the cause for rise in cancer in western society and possible solutions. Multiple researches have shown a link between animal based protein and cancer. Still other research has revealed a correlation between cancer and the amount of fiber, and sugar consumed. Others have revealed a connection between cancer and dietary intake of hormone containing products. There has also been an increase concern regarding the connection of antibiotics and cancer. In this article we will explore the evidence of these findings and possible solutions.

The introduction GMO (Genetically Modified foods) foods in the market have developed an increase concern to the concerned general public. Gmosare foods which have had their genes genetically modified (changed by science). Specific foods selected which we will explore later, for example soy beans have been genetically altered with micro-organisms such as bacteria, yeast, fish, insects etc. In GMO the DNA of the selected crop or mammal is altered with the gene splicing techniques. Immune deficiency is another problem discovered among those consuming GM foods. Multiple studies shows increase asthma, inflammation and allergies.

ABSTRACT / SUMMARY

Returning to the Old Landmark of Disease Approach

The amazing discovery of plant phytochemical has brought about an increase hope in cancer research. Phytochemicals are chemical compounds found in plant foods. These give the plants its color. These phytochemicals function as antioxidants in the system. Scientist predict that there are at least 10,000 different phytochemical which have an effect in cancer, stroke and countless other diseases. Laboratory test have shown that the mitochondria of cancer cells exposed to phytochemicals becomes inoperative. The mitochondria are the energy-producing part of the cell.

Exercise has been shown to play an important role in cancer prevention. The nurses' health study showed that woman who had 1 or more hour's daily exercise had a 30% lower risk of colon cancer than women who had less exercise. Exercise was also found to protect against breast cancer. Lifestyle influences one's risk that promotes cancerous cell growth.

The alarming rise in cancer in western society has led to a great concern. Many Americans are becoming more health conscience. Many are turning to a plant base diet to fight this dreadful disease. The Adventist mortality study showed a lower percent of cancer rate among Adventist (who are primarily vegetarian). Among the Adventist it is shown that in addition to vegetarian diet they follow a life style of daily exercise, increase water intake, increase fresh air and sunshine.

The connection between cancer and animal protein, bacteria, sugar and refined foods is indisputable. From the many researches available we can see clearly that lifestyle changes are imperative to win the cancer battle. A vegetarian lifestyle is irrefutable. We can also see that without a doubt the fascinating effect of phytochemicals on human cells in the fight against cancer. It is beneficial to us to continue to study the cause, effects of the consequences our choices make in our battle against cancer.

It is an amazing fact that, with the help of God, the body can heal itself. It is normal for a person to be well, eat the right food in the proper amount, and have the energy to work hard. The body has natural built-in ways to process the food into the needed energy. But when that individual becomes ill, the body also has natural built-in ways to produce healing. When disease strikes, the regular functions of the system are temporarily set aside and the body goes to work to regenerate itself. The body, in time of illness does not use energy for food digestion and muscular activity, it switches over to, repair, and rebuilding, cleansing. Illness causes the organs of the system to become overloaded with toxins. The disease process is the result of the body's attempt to eliminate toxins from the system and restore health.

Wholesome food for the person who is impaired in health consists of fresh, raw, fruit juices and fresh, raw, vegetable juices. This is a juice diet. Giving the patient three or four times a day, a glass of fresh raw juice is healing. It may be fruit juice or it may be vegetable juice given in different times not mixed together. Sometimes it may be a fruit-vegetable juice. The best fruits are citrus or pineapple. The best vegetables are carrots, beets, and/or celery. These are "salad vegetables." The best fruit-vegetable combination juice is carrot and apple. This enables the body to cleanse itself of retained wastes.

Other methods that can be used to hasten the healing process is the used of herbs. The use of herbs has increased since the 20th century in the US. One problem with herbs is that few of us can afford to keep more than a small collection of them on hand. Since they are not used a lot, purchasing could be a problem, since they are likely to spoil before we used them up. Another method of dealing with disease is the use of poultices which have the ability to draw poison from the system and locally. A list of popular herbs and their uses can be found in.

Massage was probably one of the earliest forms of therapy used to relieve pain and discomfort; it is natural to all of us to touch or rub a part of our body which hurts. Massage, skillfully given can bring relaxation and relief from stress. It has positive effects which help relieve pain and suffering and promote healing. We have used this tool many times both at home and in other countries. It requires no tools or equipment, no money, only a little time, and can be done anywhere.Massage produces psychological and physiological benefits. Physically, massage increases metabolism, relaxes and refreshes the muscles, hastens healing, and improves the detoxifying functions of the lymphatic system. Massage helps to prevent and relieve muscle cramps and spasms. It also improves circulation of blood and lymph, thereby improving the delivery of oxygen and nutrients to the cells as it enhances the removal of wastes. Since blood carries nutrients to the skin, massage is beneficial in keeping the skin functioning in a normal, healthy manner. Massage therapy helps in pain management.

The public has become greatly puzzled regarding the increase episodes of disease despite increase technology. Millions of dollars are spent yearly in research attempting to discover new cures for disease without success. Still millions more are spent on health insurance and EMS services. New drugs are being produced yearly to control disease with no success. The conclusion is that medicinal drugs never cure disease, but simply camouflage the symptoms for it to only reappear at a future date. Many have died from the use of medicinal drugs, yet many are suffering from the side effects that these drugs produce. Nature is constantly attempting to rid the body of accumulated toxins; the use of drugs inhibits the system from ridding itself of impurities. The general public needs to be educated regarding the change of lifestyle for the cure of disease. In this article we will explore some alternate ways of dealing with disease.

The most important element for life on this planet is air; it is the life giving and vital to survival of every living thing on this planet. Man will die within minutes without air. Air supply must be unpolluted and fresh in order to be of benefit. Study have proven the benefit of night fresh air (air circulating in room at night), this invigorates the system and provides health and proper rest. Scientist already knows that tobacco fumes, agriculture sprays, insecticides pollute air and induces disease and is harmful to both adults and children. The use of certain drugs decreases the oxygen level in the system, one such medication is aspiration, which produces hyperventilation which lowers the oxygen blood level and increase the carbon dioxide level. Homes should not have shrubbery or lots of trees around the house, for they inhibit air fresh air from circulating freely. Factory pollutants and smog produced by motor vehicle fumes; which inhaled causes red blood cells destruction. Research have proven the detrimental effect of impure air which includes liver and lung disease, frequent upper respiratory infection and frequent colds.

Another disease preventive health practice is the exposure of sunlight. Sunlight is essential to the survival of every living thing on this planet. Sunshine is one of the greatest miracle cure provided by our creator. When skin is exposed to sunshine tiny oil glands under the skin (sterols), which contain substances called ergosterols are transformed into vitamin D. Vitamin D is essential for strong bones, nails and teeth. Research have shown that sunlight destroy bacteria, lowers blood pressure, lowers cholesterol, lowers blood sugar levels, and increase white blood cell count. Sunlight has been found to increase blood's ability to carry oxygen. Sunlight increases adrenalin and calms the nerve and is beneficial to those who suffer from stress. Research has proven that sun exposure reduces hardening of the artery of the brain and improves memory. Research has shown to improve wound healing.

Water is the most power healing element on this planet. Approximately 60% of the body is water. We filter roughly 50 gallons of water daily through our kidneys and lose 2-4 quarts daily through respiration, skin and urine. Lack of water drinking causes thickening of the blood and causes a decrease in nutrient circulation to the cells. Research had proven that chlorinated water produces atherosclerosis.

Furthermore the body depends on water in order to maintain proper chemical balance which is needed for hormonal and digestive substance function.

The benefit of regular exercise has been proven over and over again by the scientific community. Our blood vessels are lined by smooth muscle and without proper exercise they begin to atrophy. Exercise increases the heart rate and blood circulation which causes exercise of the blood vessels' smooth muscles. Exercise tones the entire system and counteracts disease and fatigue. Other body functions that benefit from exercise are the voluntary muscles, digestive tract and uterus. More and more physicians are now prescribing regular exercise for their patients to promote a quicker recovery time: including post-surgical patients. Regular exercises have been proven to prevent clots, kidney stone, embolus, bone diseases and heart disease. Exercise also decreases blood cholesterol levels. Regular exercise induces a feeling of wellbeing is beneficial to fight against depression and stress.

Most disease is induced as a result of nutritional deficiency. Study have shown that those who live on meat base diet have a lower life span and suffer more from disease not seen in those who eat a plant base diet. A diet consisting of a variety of fruits, grains, vegetables, seeds and nuts provides the system with the proper nutrients necessary for proper body function. Loma Linda University has done over 700 researches showing the beneficial effects of a vegetarian diet. These researches have shown a decrease a lower risk of chronic illnesses among those whose eat a plant base diet. These researches have also revealed a lower risk in dementia among those who eat a plant base diet, especially Alzheimer's disease.

The practice of abstemiousness toward improvement of health has been greatly ignored. The use of tobacco, caffeine, soft drinks, processed food, and the use of tobacco have all contributed to a degradation of health. It will do well for one to abstain from all that is potentially harmful to the system. The use of greasy foods which is well known to clog arteries and promote heart disease is another factor which needs to abstain from.

The most important health beneficial factor is trust in divine power. We are created beings. Instructions were given us in the Bible as to how to care for the body we are privileged with. We can obey all the other 8 laws mentioned above and reap some benefits, but without trust in divine power our mind are troubled and stress itself have been proven to cause disease as revealed by countless researches. Research has shown that those who have faith in God and prayed regularly suffer less from diseases, and recuperated faster after surgical procedures.

PART ONE
BODY SYSTEMS-THEIR FUNCTIONS AND THERAPY

CIRCULATORY SYSTEM

Foods- alfalfa sprouts, brewer's yeast, garlic, wheat germ , rice polishing, liquid chlorophyll, buckwheat, sun dried olives, watercress,

Drinks- blackberry/ parsley juice, black fig juice, watercress; parsley/ grape juice; hawthorn berry tea

Vitamins- B-complex, b6 , niacin, B12, C, E bioflavonoids, folic acid, choline, inositol, pangamic acid

Minerals- calcium, iron, silicon, cobalt copper , mg, P, K, Z, manganese, N, FL, S

Herbs- hawthorn berry, ginger, garlic, cayenne, pokeroot, sassafras, burdock, chaparral, Echinacea, red clover, oat straw

DIGESTIVE SYSTEM

Foods- papaya, liquid chlorophyll, spinach, sun-dried olives, chard, celery, kale, beet greens, shredded wheat, watercress

Drinks-parsley juice, papaya juice, chlorophyll , carrot juice, potatoes peeling broth

Vitamins- A,C,B-complex, B-1,2,6,12, D,E,F,K, folic acid, inositol, niacin, pantothenic acid

Minerals- sodium, chlorine, magnesium, potassium, iron, sulphur, copper, silicon, zinc, iodine

Herbs- papaya, alfalfa, aloe Vera, peppermint, slippery elm, cayenne, burdock, comfrey, ginger, fennel, anise

GLANDULAR SYSTEM

Foods- sea vegetable, kelp, dulse, Swiss chard, turnip greens, wheat germ, lecithin, sesame seed butter, seeds and nuts

Drinks- pineapple juice, wheat germ, dulse drink, black cherry concentrate/ chlorophyll

Vitamins- B-complex, E,C choline, inositol, folic acid, pantothenic acid

Minerals- iodine, silicon, phosphorus, calcium, chlorine, magnesium, sodium, potassium, sulphur, iron, manganese

Herbs- kelp, dulse, ginseng, dong quai, licorice, Echinacea, goldenseal, dandelion

ELIMENTARY SYSTEM	INTERGLUMENTARY SYSTEM	LYMPHATIC SYSTEM
Foods- all squash, flax seed, green and yellow vegetables, alfalfa tablets, acidophilus, bran, grapes, psyllium seed, berries, sprouts, yellow cornmeal	Foods- rye, avocado, sea vegetables, apples, cucumber, millet, rice polishing, rice bran and concentrates and sprouts	**Foods**- green leafy vegetables, watercress, celery, okra, apples
Drinks- chlorophyll, coconut milk, carrot juice celery, parsley, spinach, carrot juice; flax seed tea; black cherry juice	**Drinks**- carrot/ celery/ lemon juice; cucumber/ endive/ pineapple juice	**Drinks**- potatoes peeling broth, celery juice; blue violet tea, parsley, carrot, apple juice
Vitamins- A,F , choline, B-complex, B, B2, B6, B12, C, E, inositol, niacin, folic acid, pantothenic acid	**Vitamins**- panthotenic acid, PABA, D,A, B-complex, B 2,6, 12, 1 , C, E, K, biotin, choline, folic acid, niacin, bioflavonoids	**Vitamins**-A,C choline, B-complex, B1, 2, 6, biotin, panthotenic acid, folic acid
Minerals- MG, K, NA, S , CA, chlorine, FE, PH	**Minerals**- silicon, calcium, fluorine, iron, phosphorus, potassium, sodium, sulphur, iodine, copper, manganese, zinc, magnesium	**Minerals**- potassium, chlorine, sodium
Herbs- psyllium seed, ale Vera, cayenne. Black walnut, flaxseed, comfrey, slippery elm, cascara sagrada, sena, barberry, goldenseal	**Herbs**-oat straw, shave grass, horsetail, comfrey, aloe Vera, burdock	**Herbs**- blue violet tea(leaves), chaparral, burdock , echenesea, blue flag, poke root, goldenseal, cayenne, mullein, black walnut

MUSCULAR SYSTEM	NERVOUS SYSTEM	RESPIRATORY SYSTEM
Foods-olives, rye, lima beans, rice bran, bananas, sprouts, watercress, grains, legumes, apples	**Foods**- kale, celery, rice polishing, tryptophan, brewers and nutritional yeast	**Foods**- garlic, onion, leeks, turnips, grapes, pineapple, honey(eucalyptus), green leafy vegetables
Drinks- potatoes peeling broth, dried olive tea, nut milk drink with liquid chlorophyll	**Drinks**- celery/ carrot/ prune juice; prune juice/ rice polishing, 1 tsp sesame, sunflower, or almond butter, 1 tsp honey, sliver of avocado, black cherry juice	**Drinks**- celery/ papaya juice, carrot juice watercress/ apple juice with ¼ tsp of cream of tartar; rose hip tea
Vitamins-B6, D, E, A B-complex, B12, C, biotin, choline, iron, silicon	**Vitamins**-b- complex, A, B1, B2, B6, B12, B13, C, D, E, F, choline, folic acid, inositol, niacin, pantothenic acid, pangamic acid	**Vitamins**- A,C,D, B- complex, B12, E, F, inositol, choline, bioflavonoids, folic acid, niacin, pangamic acid, pantothenic acid
Minerals- calcium, potassium, magnesium, nitrogen, chlorine, iron, silicon	**Minerals**- C, PH, MG, K ,Z, F, silicon	**Minerals**- calcium, iron, silicon, manganese, potassium, copper, fluorine
Herbs- juniper berries, rosemary, tansy, black willow, horse radish, wild cabbage, kelp, dulse, watercress, horsetail, black walnut	**Herbs**- valerian, hops, skullcap, lobelia, lady's slippers	**Herbs**- mullein, elderflowers, peppermint, yarrow lobelia, comfrey, cayenne, marshmallow, sage, coltsfoot
		Formula-(sore throat, asthma, bronchitis all lung problems, wheezing, fluids in lung)
		1/2 cup horseradish, ½ cup chopped onion, ½ cup chopped garlic, ½ tsp cayenne, 1/3tsp. Peppermint oil, 1 cup honey, ½ cup fructose- mix and take (1/2 tsp as needed
		Mix 1 cup boiled honey and ½ tsp. Peppermint oil, ½ tsp. Eucalyptus oil, 1/3 tsp. Clove oil, licorice root powder, and cayenne to tast

REPRODUCTIVE SYSTEM	SKELETAL SYSTEM	URINARY SYSTEM
Foods- sesame seeds, pumpkin seeds, seeds and nut butter, lecithin,	**Foods**- sesame seed, kale, millet, celery, barley, okra, almond, collards, turnip greens	**Foods**-watermelon (including seeds) pomegranate, apples, asparagus, liquid chlorophyll, parsley, cranberry, green leafy vegetables
Drinks- black cherry concentrate/ chlorophyll; pineapple juice, wheat germ/ dulse drink; ¾ cup carrot juice/ ¼ cup coconut milk/ 1 tbs. Wheat germ oil/ 1 tsp rice polish drink	High calcium foods vegetables (specially green leafy) carrot juice, broccoli, sesame seeds high calcium foods- brown rice, kale, turnips, spirilina, almonds, parsley-greens, pinto beans, collard greens.Almonds, amaranth and quinoa, *millet -seaweeds (nova scotia dulse, Norwegian kelp) wheat grass juice, green drinks -garlic and onions are needed for healthy bones because of the sulfur -flaxseed oil (if you are eating a good diet, then distilled water is best to drink)	**Drinks**- celery/ pomegranate juice; black currant juice/ juniper berry tea; pomegranate juice; celery, parsley, asparagus; beet juice, grapes
Vitamins- B-complex, E, A, B2, B6, C, D, F		**Vitamins**- A,B-complex, b2, 6, C, D, E, choline, panthotenic acid
Minerals; zinc, calcium, iodine, phosphorus, iron, sodium, chlorine, potassium, fluorine, silicon		**Minerals**- CA, K, manganese, , chlorine, MG
Herbs- black cohosh, licorice, dong quai, ginseng, blessed thistle, blue cohosh, uvaursi, raspberry, squaw vine, chickweed, saw palmetto, false unicorn, raspberry	**Drinks**-black mission figs, black cherry juice, green kale juice, celery/ parsley juice	**Herbs**- juniper berries, uvaursi, parsley, goldenseal, slippery elm, elder flowers, ginger, dandelion, buchu marshmallow
	Vitamins; C,D, A, B-complex, b2, b6, b12, E, F, folic acid, niacin, pantothenic acid, bioflavonoids	
	Minerals- calcium, fluoride, copper, manganese, iron, iodine, sulphur, zinc, silicon, phosphorus, potassium, sodium	
	Herbs- comfrey, kale, alfalfa, boneset, poke root, chicory, juniper berries, arnica, flowers, elder flowers, oat straw, alfalfa, Irish moss	

PART TWO
DISEASE AND TREATMENT SUGGESTIONS

ABDOMINAL PAIN	
Catnip, hops/ valerian teas (3x daily) **Heating pad**- hot water bottle and fomentations to the abdomen. **Enemas** -lukewarm tap water	**Moist heat** - severe cases hot applications for an hour, removed for an hour and applied again for an hour throughout the day.
ABSCESSES, SORES, BOIL	
Barley green known to cure boils **Apply** -*honey* externally to the area. -*chlorophyll* water to the area several times a day will keep it cleansed -Charcoal-3 tbsp. Charcoal + 2 tbs. Flaxseed + 1/2 tbsp. Castor oil- mix-put on cloth - heat up and apply. -*formula*-2 oz. Powdered myrrh+ 1oz. Goldenseal+ 1/2 oz. Cayenne +1oz. Peppermint oil –mix with 70 % alcohol let stand for 7 days shaking daily - apply -*figs* preheat and apply, overnight or split a fig heat and apply hot - *t-tree oil* -*poultice* of raw potato mixed with flaxseed. / *wet cabbage*/ onions, -*apply*- lemon- vitamin-e goldenseal or -slippery elm 1 tbs. + baking yeast 1 tbsp.-mix let set and apply over pain -*Apply* dressing of fresh *comfrey* leaves and root or a paste made from raw garlic on gauze for 8-10 hours. With 3% boric acid can be used or a hot Epsom salt compress -*Echinacea*, or a clay poultice. -*flaxseed* poultice to soften and mature the head. -*slippery elm* bark and lobelia poultice soothes and helps promote healing. **Hot compresses** or ice bags -relieve the pain; + promote healing.	**Boil-Apply moist heat** - itchy, mild pain, local swelling- red inflamed, filled with pus (clean towel, cloth, or gauze that is wet in warm water) 3-4 times daily to the boil. It will reduce pain and help bring it to a head more quickly. Avoid irritating the area it will spreading the pus. Avoid exercise which might cause sweating until it heals. **Open skin ulcers**- place herbal poultices, such as German chamomile, marigold, arnica, euphorbia, cliff rose, snake root, and/or witch hazel. Red clover tea and carrot and beet juice. Burdock root, cayenne, and yellow dock root. **Sores that won't heal**: vitamin E:200 units a day **Drink** distilled water with fresh lemon juice -1/2 tbsp. Ginger +3 tbsp. Charcoal, for 1 week; Echinacea tea, 3 cups daily; silver biotin **Vitamin/ minerals-**_zinc (proven to help_; vitamin C orally to bowel tolerance, along with A, B complex, and E. Take -take garlic 1-3 times daily **Herbs-** comfrey, red clover blossoms, yellow dock root, chickweed, plantain, and wild cherry bark, oat straw, goldenseal, dandelion, and burdock root.

ACID REFLUX (heartburn)	
Drink some raw potato juice. Whiz up an unpeeled potato and drink it down	<u>**Immediately**</u> drink a large glass of water **Drink lemon** water
ACNE	
Bad facial acne- linked to facial parasites- check potassium deficiency -zinc clears acne **Apply- poultice:** chaparral, dandelion, yellow dock root-watercress leaves to area -sap of wild lettuce -rub lemon juice to area -white clay /Swedish bitters -apply 1 part apple cider with 10 parts water -Apply cool cooked oatmeal and milk or cooked -carrots or ripe tomatoes blended with 1 tbs. -oatmeal and 1 tsp. Lemon juice -Black walnut tincture/-put on aloe Vera -tea compresses applied hot or cold (witch hazel /goldenseal /ephedra/ mullein/ slippery elm/ and white oak bark / golden seal/ t-tree/ calendula) -Honey -black strap molasses (rub at night and wash of in a.m.)	**Hot Epson salt bath** with about 2-3 lb. Epson salt in the water/salt glow **Scars-acne scars:-**place fresh pineapple on scars and take bromelein 750mg daily steam to face -with eucalyptus+ red clover+ strawberry leaf and lavender **Detox herbs-**cleaver- excellent for the complexion-apply to skin, Echinacea, chaparral, comfrey, tree, dandelion, alfalfa, red clover, kalala leaves **Formula:-**2p red clover+ 1 p each- Echinacea, nettles, dandelion, burdock+ ½ p licorice (place in #00 cap take 3-4 3x daily) **Take-**zinc supplements proven to clear acne -take clay orally, mix 1 tbs. In 8 oz. Of water 2x daily and apply clay mask 2x/day **Take steam baths**
ADHD	
Supplement-St. John's worth, grape seed extract, valerian root (works well)- 4 cap 2x daily, wild lettuce 3x daily, passion flower (hysteria in children) Vitamin-b complex 300mg daily =*best*	**Supplement-** calcium 1000mg daily , 5 HTP, zinc, carrot juice 8oz daily; vegetable juice 3x daily, manipol, vitamin- b6, thiamine, pantothenic acid folic acid flax oil- 4 tsp daily, beta carotene, vitamin-c, e calcium magnesium
ADENOID	
Three times a day, give herb teas such as red clover, sassafras, and burdock root.	**Gargle several** times a day with goldenseal tea. **Echinacea and myrrh** are very good for all glandular swellings.
ADDICTION	
Take 1 tsp. Black strap molasses 3x daily -1 tsp of carob in 1 cup of hot water, take before bedtime -4 charcoal tab 2 times daily **Cabbage juice** drink 1 pint daily -noni **Charcoal-** 1 tsp in six ounces of water 3x daily	**Formula-**together- 1 cup honey- 2 tsp. Peppermint powder,1/3 tsp peppermint tincture- 1/3 tsp. Spearmint tincture- 1 tsp. Liquid smoke,1 tsp. Cayenne pepper- 4 lemon juiced-take ½ tsp. Every hour and as needed

Black strap molasses take 1 tsp. 3x daily -give 1 enema 2x daily

Delirium tremors:-quassia chip tea

Use laxative herbs to keep the bowels open -give lobelia and bayberry bark as an emetic to empty the stomach- repeat until empty

Drastic-treatment:-club moss (lycopodium variety)-boil in water for 20 minutes drink a full glass of this liquid then immediately a full glass of vodka this will (causes immediate painful vomit)do this 2-3 times 1 after another (this causes a permanent allergy (vomit with alcohol)

Formulas: 1p = 1 part = 1 tbs. -1p vervain , 1p skullcap- 3p hops , 1p valerian, 1/2p cayenne, 3p peppermint- 1p catnip- mix and use 2 tab. Per 1 cup of hot water and steep for 30 minutes- take 1 cup 3 times per day

Formula: -mix 1 part apple juice, 1 tsp. Cayenne- 2 drops clove oil, 4 oz. Apple cider vinegar, 1/2 tsp ginger oil, 1/2 cup- honey. Take 1 tsp as needed

Vitamin c (5,000-25,000 mg) in divided doses daily-eat candy bar instead of tobacco-extra calcium and chamomile (3-6 times daily)-B-complex vitamins

Drink 3 qtrs. Water daily

Give 1 enema 2 x daily.

2high enema daily with teas of bayberry bark/ red raspberry leaves

Neutral bath-for 2-3 hours- keep head and neck cool give teas while in the bath (such as catnip, skullcap, peppermint, spearmint, valerian, gentian, sweet balm, +/ calamus -1 tsp. Of herb per 1 cup of water only)-several times while in the bathtub-give a small cold shower- give a brisk salt glow right before finishing, place the patient back in the warm water to warm up then give a final cold shower or rub- dry thoroughly- put him to bed

Wet sheet pack nightly /salt glow daily/ hot bath nightly/ steam bath daily

Smokers-lick on licorice sticks / raw carrots with cravings

ADRENAL

Description-The systolic is the first number in a blood pressure reading, and the diastolic is the second. For example, 120/80. The systolic should be *10 points higher* when you are standing than when you are lying down.

Lie down and rest for 5 minutes, and then have someone take your blood pressure. Then stand up and take it immediately again. The blood pressure will probably be somewhat higher**.**
If it is lower when standing than when lying flat, the adrenals are not working properly. The lower it is, the worse the condition of the adrenals

Licorice root can be used as a supplement in tablets, capsules, extract, or as a tea.

Herbal-a=acute; sa=subacute; c=chronic; d=degenerative

A-(hyperactive) ephedra, valerian, blue skullcap

Sa- (hypoactive) ephedra, buchu leaves, cayenne

C-(Adison's disease, chronic insufficiency) chaparral, buchu leaves, cayenne

D-(degenerative stage) Echinacea, chaparral, goldenseal

Herbs-goat weeds -chaparral -blueberry leaf tea (6 tsp. Per qt. Water steep for 10 minutes)- drink 2 cups daily -psyllium powder 1 tbsp. In glass water / juice -kelp dulse/ Norwegian kelp -about 4-6 tabs 3x daily -black walnut 2 capsules 2x daily for 2 weeks and 1 weeks off- then 3 capsules 2x daily for 2 weeks

AIDS (acquires immune deficiency syndrome)

Some use this only (KYOLIC GARLIC 10 X 14 DAYS THAN INCREASE TO 20 QD)- till healed

Research:- professional injection research blood-root and celandine improve after 20 days-aged

Supplement from whole foods:-vitamin- mineral (specially -E)-vitamin-A, B complex, C bioflavo-noids, selenium, zinc, potassium, calcium, magnesium -flaxseed oil 4,000-6,000 mg daily garlic preparations significantly help-licorice root was found to help

TAKE- general treatments:- poke root - 1 tbsp. In 8 oz. Of water take 4x per day- pau d'arco 10 capsules daily- aloe Vera concentrate- 1/2 cup daily -eliminates aids virus -noni

- cleanse formula(see cleanse summary) one tablespoons 3x daily

-make tea- 3tbs each of peach leaf, yarrow, blue vervain, put all in 2 qt. Of hot water 4cup daily- take bloodroot, celandine, aged garlic and licorice

Rebuild the immune system:-burdock , garlic, goldenseal, pau d'arco, psyllium, suma, -ginkgo, garlic, black radish, dandelion root, silymarin, -aloe Vera, kelp -St. John's wort -aloe Vera inhibit the growth and spread of HIV

APPLY- castor oil packs –this will increase WBC and RBC

DIET- diet: -lots of broccoli -Brussels sprouts, cabbage- raw foods -drink 3 glass carrot juice daily

ALLERGY

Check for parasites/ toxic release/ need fix digestive tract lining

Pulse test

-*description*: a home method to determine which foods you are allergic to.

Each test must be continued for a period of time to be effective

-*procedure*: take pulse before eating anything- each 1 food and check pulse 15 minutes later and 30 min. Then in 60 minutes-if you pulse is 10 beats higher than the pulse rate before you ate then you are allergic to that food

-*other test:* eliminate several foods from your diet for several days- do this for a month or two then gradually add these foods to your diet and do pulse test-you may also fast for 5 days then gradually add foods to diet doing pulse test-keep an ongoing diary of foods and pulse test results

Six charcoal tablets (or 3 capsules or 1 heaping teaspoon of charcoal powder stirred in a glass of water) take three times daily in the mid-morning, mid-afternoon, and at bedtime for two weeks

Diet-eat three to four olives with each meal for about three weeks.

Eye redness- drink hot mullein flower tea

Formula:-alfalfa 1 tbs.+ ½ tbs. Yellow dock, 1 tbsp. Chickweed, chaparral 1 tbs. Echinacea 2 tbs. Pau D'Arcy 2 tbs. Kelp ½ tbs. Black cohosh 1 tbs. Mix and take 4 capsules 3x daily-blood purify for allergies- red clover 2 tsp., burdock 2 tsp., yellow dock 1 tsp.

Congested- drink hot red clover or nettles tea

Hay fever severe - cold application to the forehead-replace when it begins to get warm- keep it on for 3-4 hours even after you are feeling better in one hour

Irritated mucus membrane: thyme , hyssop, marjoram, or lavender

Itchy eyes: cold compress of witch hazel diluted in 4 parts boiling water

Mucus-for excess mucus- nettle, ephedra, osha, eyebright, yerra, mansa, bayberry, evening primrose oil

Nasal and respiratory symptoms-asthma etc.- stinging nettle1/2 tsp. Tincture/ 1-2 caps. Every 2-4 hours-wild yam, horseradish, feverfew, dandelion, goldenseal, comfrey, fenugreek, lobelia, Echinacea

Postnasal drip:-flush nose with salt water and use a bulb syringe and flush nostril with salt water -herb tea with lemon and honey

-room humidifier -fruit fast -take a few enemas

Hot foot bath- for nasal congestion

Hot compress-directly to the face. Squeeze a towel from hot water and apply it directly over the sinus areas for five minutes at the end of that time, place a towel that has been squeezed from ice cold water or cold tap water over the area for thirty seconds. Continue alternating hot and cold for three changes, ending with the cold. After each remedy the person should lie in bed 30 minutes repeat the treatment four times daily

Immune system to stimulate - Echinacea 1/2- 1 tsp. Tincture , (3-4 times daily for 1 week) **Chemical allergy:** -vitamin-a, b- complex, grape seed extract -zinc, copper, vitamin-c	for the first week and once daily thereafter until sinusitis has cleared
ALZHEIMER	
Blueberry fast reverse it **Herbs:** helpful herbal remedies include ginkgo, hawthorn berry tea, ginseng, and Mistletoe. - Chinese common club moss*, ging-ko Bilbao -Asian / Siberian ginseng -astralagus -St. John's wort - ginger -rosemary -club moss -horse balm	-blackstrap molasses, lecithin -flax oil (1 tbs. Daily) -lecithin 1 tsp. 2x daily -rosemary, horse balm, club moss, choline, black strap molasses Oil very important (grape seed oil, linseed, vita-min e oil)- take 2 tbs. 3x daily -brewer's yeast 1 tbsp. Daily in juice
ANEMIA	
Check copper, b12- deficiency, parasites- can cause pernicious anemia, vitamins prevents ane-mia, need a cleanse **Severe**- Drink about four ounces of grape juice with an egg once a day for three days. **Beet & yellow dock;** apricots **Blend-** wheat grass, beets, molasses= blood transfusion **Sun bathing** **Wet sheet pack** (neutral stage) **Formula Anemia** -drink the following for 30 days -1 gallon of grape juice +1cup raisins+1 cup apricots+1cup figs+1/2cup black strap molasses+5 tsp blackberry extract let sit overnight on counter-refrigerate after 10 hours take 4 oz. 3-4x daily **Formula**-blend and take 1cup three times daily of: grape juice 1 gallon+ apricots 1/3 cups figs 1/3 cups+ molasses 1 cup+ raisins 1/3 cups-leave in jar overnight take 4 oz. 3x daily	**Formula**: mix 1 cup each- blackstrap molasses, figs, prunes, raisins, and apricots in large bottle of grape juice- let sit for 24 hours -refrigerate and drink 4 oz. 2x daily **Formula:** 2 cups pineapple juice + 1 cup fresh parsley or 1 cup fresh dandelion greens-blend till smooth and drink daily **Formula**: 1 tsp. Bilberry/ chickweed tea to 1 cup boiling water- remove from heat and steep for 15- 20 minutes- drink 2x daily **Cold mitten rub**-short cold baths-to stimulate the bone marrow and the circulation, adjusts the temperature of the water in the tub between 40 and 90 degrees. The greater the cold, the less time spent. Try ½ minute at 40 – 50 degrees, 1 minute at 60-70 degrees, 2 minutes at 70-80 degrees, 3 minutes at 80-85 degrees, and 3 ½ minutes at 90 degrees.
ANGINA PECTORIS (chest pain)	
Symptom:-recurrent pain beneath the sternum -it last for 30-60 seconds-it is a severe constricting pain in the chest, often radiating from the heart to theleft shoulder and down to the arm **Mix** one cup soy sprouts, cooked. Add 5000mg vitamin-c and 1/3 cup rose hips. Mix in raw veg-etables eat 1 cup or more daily	**Take 1 capsule cayenne** pepper 3x daily, 4 cap-sules Hawthorne 3x daily **Formula:** - mix 1 tsp. Lecithin (a natural fat emul-sifier) + 400 iu. Vitamin e with 4 tbs. Pumpkin seeds, one banana and 8 ounces soy milk- blend drink daily

Drink 10 ounces carrot juice 3 x daily add 4 ounces green drink juice and ½ tsp. Kelp-drink garlic tea, add peeling from grapefruits, and peeling from lemons. Add a large onion, 2 tsp. Pectin, ½ tsp. Cayenne pepper, 3 blended onion bulbs, 2 blended garlic bulbs, 5 tbs. Yarrow, mix in 1 qt. Of water, boiling for 10 minutes

Herbs:-hawthorn 4 capsules 3x daily, angelica, ginger, garlic, bilberry, purslane-ginseng extract -rosemary- cause kidneys reduce edema

Grape seed extract - lowers blood pressure which can help heart disease

Hot arm baths 40°c degrees (104°f) for about 5 minutes.-often relieve pain immediately.

APPENDIX

If there is a most terrible pain, rush the person to the hospital at once. If you wait beyond that point, he may die.-**Do not swallow laxatives or laxative herbs. This can cause the appendix to rupture!**

Symptom: pain and tenderness in the lower right quadrant of the abdomen, vomiting, low- high-grade fever pain may be worse with coughing, pressure, rigidity of the abdominalmuscles there may be pain that is worse around navel

Diet-fast

Herbs-a=acute; **sa**=subacute; **c**=chronic; **d**=degenerative

A-(appendicitis) slippery elm, uvaursi, blue violet, cayenne, goldenseal

Sa-(catarrhal) cascara sagrada, blue violet, cayenne, goldenseal

C-(chronic inflammation) cayenne, goldenseal, chaparral

D- (degenerative stage) cayenne, goldenseal, Echinacea, chaparral

Formula: make and drink a tea made with the following- vervain, plantain, goldenseal, flax seed,chickweed, nettle, lobelia, mint, oregano, mix all take 3 cups daily-*buckthorn bark

Formula: mix together 1cup charcoal +1/2 cup of honey - take 1 tsp every hour till mixture is gone

Drink small amounts ofwater every so often.

Do not eat too much at a time enema:1/2 quart enema 2x daily-use very warm *enema*mild*

Do not do hot and cold shower- do-cold to pain area and hot to legs and hips-do not apply heat over area - will swell and burst

Do foot massage

Ice cap or ice bag (about one-half full of finely chopped ice) on the naval. This will draw inflammation away from the appendix - placing hot packs on a distant area. A hot Hip-and-Leg Pack is applied, plus placing an ice bag on the appendix

Castor oilfor chronic cases only

Include 1 tsp. Psyllium in juice or water, 3 times a day, for 2 weeks after the appendicitis has ceased. **Laxatives:** aloes two # 2 capsules daily

APPETITE

Can't eat:-rectal bolus-add desired herb -pour coconut oil/ coco butter/ slippery elmover powdered herbs - to dough consistent roll let sit for 30 minutes andfreeze and used as suppository (use every 2 days 3x per week-slippery elm tea-6-8 oz. Retention enema

Drink**-**alfalfa tea, coconut water,

Alfalfa tea recipe-cook does not boil, in a glass/ enamel pan, use 1 oz. Of untreated seed (such as use in sprouting) with 1 ¼ pt. Water. Keep water moving but not boiling for ½ hour, cool and squeeze seeds for more water, refrigerate for no more than 1 day. Mixthe strong base with = amounts of water (drink 6-7 cups daily for at

Loss appetite: Swedish bitters, vitamin b-1- coconut water has plenty nutrients-slippery elm tea –nutritious- lemon water- dandelion tea-	least 2weeks) alfalfa tea **Retention enema**-after colon cleanse of 1 tbs. Acidophilus +8 oz. Warm water and inject
	Herbs: gentian, angelica, goldenseal, ginger, marjoram*

ARTERIOSCLEROSIS (arteries)

Silicon decreases atherosclerosis and - arteriosclerosis- needed by the arterial walls- copper, manganese keeps coronary arteries strong- valadium	**Needed for arteries**- advance formula- see phone number above (vitamin-c, alpha lipoic acid,vitamin b5, gugulipid, garlic, bromelain, vitamin-e, selenium, n-acetyl-cystine).
Garlic eaten with cholesterol foods **Eggplant** tends to lower cholesterol levels	

ARTHRITIS

study shows benefit in 85% arthritis patients when (eggplant, tomatoes, white potatoes, pepper) were eliminated from the diet	**Apply**- eucalyptus oil + water rub to area and heat
Herbs-a=acute; **sa**=subacute; **c**=chronic; **d**=degenerative	-grated raw potatoes, /castor oil /comfrey leaves tea
A-(gout, bursitis, arthritis) alfalfa, burdock, comfrey	-cayenne pepper paste -apply packs of warmed castor oil, moisture comfrey leaves, or grated potato to area- charcoal poultice to area
Sa- (rheumatism) alfalfa, chaparral, oat straw	Apply-DMSO (dimethyl sulfoxide) **pain:-**peach leaf tea 6 cups daily
C-(rheumatoid arthritis) capsicum, chaparral, black cohosh	**Pine needle** 1lb. + 1lb. Of pine cones boil for 1 hr. Let cool for 12 hours – strain and bathe in tub
D-(osteoarthritis) chaparral, black cohosh, oat straw, aloe	**Electric blankets** at night or hot packs
Drastic treatment for knee arthritis- garlic 3-4 bulbs poultice for 5-6 hours- will-form boils and pop them to remove toxins	**Local alternate bath**-acute inflammation
	Local-cold fomentation-heating compress to joint
Drink- raw potatoes with skin- drink 1st thing in the morning (dilute with 50-50 water)	**Sun bathing**
Formula -rub peppermint oil to skin before applying. Mix petroleum and cayenne and apply- with paper towel and saran wrap	**Russian steam bath**- and salt glow treatments 3x daily
	No ice massage Caution-avoid cold douche, long sweating process,
Severe arthritis pain blend 3 garlic	-warm bath
-4 cups apple cider vinegar in tub and **soak- apple cider vinegar** to area- nightly soak and cover- make vinegar hot 1st	**Hot tub bath**/ hot shower -heating pack/ pad to area (put liniment to area first) for 1 1/2- 2 hours
Herb-cayenne pills, 12 raw pecans per day , aloe gel, mandrake root #0 every night-yucca + devils	**Hot vinegar soaks**- 10oz. To tub every night-moist heat to effected area 15-30 minutes 2x daily - area inflamed and red- use bagged crushed ice

claw in pills or tea (pain relief) take one glass of grapefruit juice-daily eat alfalfa sprouts, yellow sweet clover, noni

-research in India- ginger (1 1/2-3 1/2 tsp given) more than 75% had relief

-kombucha tea, sarsaparilla -British research- shows licorice root effective

-take 3 yucca tablets with each meal or 2 prim- rose capsules 2x daily

Paraffin bath - to effected area

Alternate hot and cold to painful area

Very hot Epson salt bath (3 ½ lb. Salt)

ASTHMA

80 %of asthma is caused by allergies

Sit straight on chair breath in through nose and out through pursed lips

Lie on stomach with head and chest over edge of bed cough gently x 2-3 minutes

Adult-cayenne-stops attacks

BABY WITH ASTHMA:-give no honey until 1 1/2 years old- make a weak solution cayenne andwater in eye dropper and put under infants tongue as needed

To relax baby- hops tea and honey or catnip and honey to induce sleep- chamomile +honey - at attack feed no milk- only alfalfa tea or pepper- mint tea

Cayenne and water (weak solution) in eye drop- per on tongue-vitamin-c 1000mg

½ oz. Laxative tea (weak Senna)- enema if fever- hops tea/ catnip tea (no honey if less than 1 ½ years old)

Make a cough syrup for children (pour 1 qtr. Of water over the above herbs (no vinegar or alco- hol)- let stand x1 hour then strain- add 1 pint of honey- place over low heat let it evaporate to 2 cupful's seal in small jars

Mullein oil is excellent-in a little water

1cup of hot water + anise (specially at attach), mullein, catnip, every hour till relieved (drink while hot)

After blending a clove of garlic in a cup of wa- ter, drink it. If vomited, give another cup. The garlic really helps.

Take a cup of hot water, catnip tea, or mullein tea each hour.

Swedish bitters-(cardiac asthma)-apply compress of Swedish bitters to liver area +drink 1 cups of club moss tea + 1 tsp of Swedish bitters 2x daily am and pm

Aloe Vera- breathes in vapor from aloe Vera leaves in boiling water.

Keep the head cool by sponging with cool water or use a fan.

Pouring cold water on the back of the neck is helpful. As the person bends over, the water is poured on the back of the neck from a contain- er holding about a gallon of water. Hold it 24 inches above the neck, pour it for about 30-90 seconds. Do this 3 times a day

A vaporizer, which blows cold, moist air, is helpful during an attack. Eucalyptus or Menthol oil may be added to the water.

Rub peppermint oil over chest-

For severe air hunger in asthmatics alternate hot arm baths and hot foot baths.

Mustard plaster- heating compress to chest

-Proportions

Adult—1 part mustard to 3 or 4 parts flour

Child—1 part mustard to 8 or 10 parts flour

Infant—1 part mustard to 12 or 14 parts flour

-Apply oil to chest- apply plaster to chest, cover with flannel then plastic (stop when patient states it feels hot.)

Fever treatment- increase body temperature to 104-105 for 5-7 hours(will get relief at second treatment) or up to 3 hours

Neutral bath (94-97 f.) Up to two hours helpful -give garlic enema 3x daily

Lobelia is an herb that, when sipped slowly, relaxes the nerves and tends to stop the spasm. (If one drinks more quickly, it has a different effect, and induces vomiting.)

Tea-comfreys 2tbs. Blend in 6 oz. Veggie. Juice take 2x daily -mullein 2 tbsp. 2x daily (mix in 8 oz. Mullein in 12 oz. Hot water) make tea drink 3 cups per day

-skullcap 3 cap. 3x daily -black cohosh 1 cap. 2x daily -yarrow 3 cap 2x daily

-blessed thistle 2 cap 2x daily - peppermint tea 1 cup 2x daily

Tea- 3 parts each of coughwort, plantain, sage, mullein- use 3-4 tsp. In 1 cup boil h20

-goldenseal- ½ tsp. 2x daily -angelica (removes phlegm)- 3 cups daily

Removes phlegm -3 cups of angelica tea daily

Drastic case- 1tbs. Lobelia tincture in water (will vomit.) -lobelia tincture*

Go on a juice fast 3 days / month -angelica tea 3 cups daily

Give an emetic

Garlic enema 3x daily-

Eat lots of kiwi

Hot fomentations to the back of the neck, thorax, and front of the chest are helpful, along with a hot footbath.

Hot arm baths 40°c degrees (104°f) for about 5 minutes.

Hot Epson salt bath daily-steam bath daily/

Steam bathstake 3 weekly

Hot Epson baths 5 lbs. Of salt daily

Herbs-blue vervain, horehound, comfrey, coltsfoot, marshmallow, valerian

Formulas:-1/2 tsp. Cayenne+ 3oz. Lemon juice+1/2 tsp. Peppermint oil+2 bulbs of blended garlic+2 blended onions+2 oz. Horse radish+1/2 cup of fructose mix and take 1/2 teaspoon as needed

-mix peppermint oil + honey + cayenne+ lemon juice

Vitamin - C 10,000mg every hour for 3 day- B12 1000mg - A 25,000 2x daily

AUTOIMMUNE DISEASE

Supplement-2tbs. Daily **flax seed oil**- magnesium, purslane, poppy seeds, cow peas-black currant oil

Herbs-gingko bilboa, coenzyme q10,mthylsulfonyl-methane

Herbs-ginkgo, suma, gotu kola, kelp, chamomile, skullcap, valerian -evening primrose

Eat- blueberries, pineapple

Handle stinging nettle plants with gloves and slap it to skin/ get stung by honey bees

Hydrotherapy-sun bathing

Russian steam bath

BITES

Charcoal-in order to make a poultice for a bee sting, spider bite, or other venomous bites, dissolve a bit of charcoal powder or crunch up several charcoal tablets in plain water, changed every 15 or 20 minutes for the first hour or two-*drink charcoal water every hour till danger is passed*

Ant (fire):-baking soda, vinegar and lemon juice, white oak bark , witch hazel, plantain tea

-baking soda -make paste by adding water

-crushed plantain leaf poultice

-ice pack or cool compress -vinegar and -lemon juice-

Bees/ wasp:-remove sting -apply damp charcoal to area -place a paste of baking soda andwater to area -cold compress or ice- 6 hours later apply

Bed bugs:-sprinkle sulfur to rugs, bedding- and do not use them x 3 weeks-then shakeoff the sulfur

Spider bites

Spider (black) in a short time agonizing pain throughout the body, especially in the abdomen, which may be rigid as a board. Cold sweats, nausea, vomiting, difficulty in breathing and sometimes delirium and convulsions occur. Black widow venom is more potent, drop for drop, than the poison of a pit viper

Spider (brown recluse) -a"bull's eye" appearance of a blister encircled by red and white rings- few hours after skin around the bite becomes red and swollen-eventually most of the tissue dies- leaving a deep sore that may take months to heal (ittakes sometimes as much as five days to see symptoms), treatment had to be continued for four months.

-*If there is swelling or pain after* a spider bite, keep calm and apply a *constricting band 2-4 inches above* (above) the bite. Loosen the band for 15 seconds every 10 minutes. Do not let the extremity turn blue! Do not move the affected area, and keep it below the heart level, if possible. The victim should lie down.

-Pack ice around the wound.

Lice: - (pediculosis) Heat combs and brushes to 151° F. For 5-10 minutes; soak for an hour in 2% Lysol solution or freeze for 30 minutes.

-Launder clothing and bedding in hot water. Non-washable items should be sealed in a plastic sack for 10 days. Soak the place on the body for 30 minutes in very warm, soapy, water.

-The hair can be doused in *kerosene* and then wrapped in a towel.

- *50-50 mixture of kerosene and olive oil* can be put on the scalp to get rid of the nits.

-*Garlic compresses* can be placed on the scalp for 2 hours.

Mosquito: To relieve itching: Rub with fresh lemon juice or raw garlic; repeat as often as possible. Rub with damp salt. Rub with vitamin C tablet or powder.

Scorpion: -ammonia water -charcoal poultice

Snake bitecaution-(do not put ice- will drive the poison to heart) (do not pour alcohol - it speeds up the venom)

Do not give liquor to the person, thinking that this will help him. It does not! -cause intense pain; frequently there is nausea, vomiting, and unconsciousness.

-*Antidote*-snake antidote for snake bite**:** charcoal +/ juice of 5 lemons in a glass jar= antidote for snake bite-danger over after 2 days

-*1ˢᵗ immediately lay down x 2 hours, Keep calm and work carefully. Excitement speeds up the blood flow to the heart.*

-*apply* a tourniquet above the limb where the wound is. Tight enough to shut off the venous blood, but not so tight that it stops the arterial circulation. Loosen the band 15 seconds every 10 minutes.

-*suction the venom with mouth for 30-60 minutes* (snake venom are only poisons in blood not stomach)see spider for supplements and doses

-*give enema*

-*Wash the wound immediately with warm water and vinegar; let it dry, and then pour upon the*

Spider treatment

-*pack ice around* wound

-*chew and swallow 10 charcoal* pills and apply as a poultice

-*Drink as much yellow dock as possible or take 2 capsules every hour till symptoms recede.*

-*Swallow Echinacea.*

-*Apply white oak bark poultices;*Slippery elm, plantain, or comfrey is also good.

-*Supplements-* _Massive doses of vitamin C may save a life._ -take c(dose of 4,000 mg followed by 1,000-2,000mg every hour-reduce with diarrhea),-calcium(500 mg every 6 hours), magnesium(1,000mg),-pantothenic acid (500mg every 8 hours for 2 days)

Caterpillar: put tape to area and pull to remove hairs- then apply plantain leaves

Centipede: charcoal, cold/ ice

Chiggers:- A red spot that itches intensely for about 3 days remove them with nails / castor oil/ Vaseline apply clear nail polish to the spot -charcoal/ plantain poultice-apply clear nail polish to area to smother them -hot bath, baking soda paste-sprinkle cornstarch to area -ground oatmeal paste

Coral, stingray, sea urchin: -flush do not rub area with sea water-apply alcohol, vinegar, ammonia, alum, meat tenderizer-remove fragments -immerse area in hot water x 30 min.

_Dog-mad dog bite_*rabies **(Hydrophobia)**

-symptoms will appear within 10 days if it is rabid

-Wash the wound with water right away and then mix *with half and half vinegar* and warm water, and wash the wounds with it. When dry, apply 1-2 drops of muriatic acid (hydrochloric acid) to each wound. Do this even if, what appears to be, a rabid dog only licks a previous wound on you.

-For extra precaution, you may apply a

-tourniquet and a rubber vacuum cup

-gentian root poultice,clintonia also for -*prolonged steam bath*

wound a few drops of hydrochloric acid, and that will neutralize and destroy the poison of the saliva (If acid is not available, you may burn the wound with a magnifying glass in the sunlight. Or use a red-hot iron)

-*charcoal*- After the suction process is over- drink charcoal or take it from the campfire- 1/2 glass of water- to 1 tsp. Of charcoal drink 1 cup every 15 min till danger pass- or 10 charcoal, paste(if no charcoal apply wet mud)

-*after 2 days do steam* bath

-*Diet*-Throughout all this time, you should eat no food.

-*Kerosene-If, after several hours, the bite area is still swollen and painful, put kerosene on a cloth and applies it, keeping it wet for several hours.* This will help neutralize the poison.

-*Onion*-An alternative is to grind up raw onions and apply to the area. Leave them there until an offensive odor, not of onions, is noticed. Remove; bathe the area; and apply more raw, crushed, onions until the

-*Herb*-common catalpa, cyana [cornflower]

-drink rue- and apply to area-hyacinth bean, Venus maidenhair fern

Ticks:**LYME disease -"bull's eye"- spot** within a day a rash about 3 inches around the bite occur (10% do not develop a rash)between 2-32 days after the bite- symptoms appear- headache, nausea, fatigue, flu-like symptoms, stiffneck, backache, vomiting-ultimately enlargement of lymph nodesand spleen may occur- along with arthritis braindamage ,irregular heart rhythm, - some of and these symptoms slowly pass away after 2-3 years and may reoccur-may have a raised rash for 1-2 days/ several weeks -can develop arthritic type jointpains -70% of those who remain untreated develops central nervous system diseaseslater on

-take at least 30 sec to pull of slowly then apply crushed plantain leaves

After removal of tick: -apply aloe Vera, lemon - apply alcohol/ t-tree oil/ calendula/hydrogen peroxide/ St. John's wort / Echinacea/ goldenseal-extract

**Jelly fish:** headache, muscle cramps, coughing, shortness of breath, nauseaand vomiting; Immediately rinse the wound with salt water. Do not use fresh water, because it activates any stinging cells which have not already burst, do not rub the skin.

-Neutralize the area Use rubbing or ethyl (liquor) alcohol, vinegar, ammonia, or meat tenderizer. Apply a paste of sand and seawater; then wrap your hand in a towel and wipe them off or scrape them off with a credit card or knife

-apply aloe Vera gel / plantain tincture to area

Lice -_thyme essential_ oil 4 drops in 1 tbsp. Shampoo lather in hair and leave on for 5 minutes, rinse and put = parts warm water and vinegar to hair and cover with plastic cap for 15 minutes, comb with lice comb , repeat in 1 week if necessary

-_Hot vinegar_ (or a 50-50 vinegar/water mixture) applied to the scalp will loosen eggs, so they can be vigorously combed out of the hair with a fine-toothed comb.

- Eyebrows; Petroleum jelly has been recommended to suffocate the lice.

-Use, as a hair wash, either Labrador tea or field larkspur.

-_herbs_-take 6 echenesea capsule daily, garlic capsules (1,200 mg daily) -may have to take doxycycline

-_Supplement_-charcoal- 8 tab 3x

-other helpful herbs- red clover, pau d'arco, feverfew (do not use during pregnancy), licorice, dandelion tea - drink as much peppermint teas as possible-Echinacea, yucca, and goldenseal

-b-complex vitamins (500-1,000mg), 3x daily -E (400-800 iu. Daily)

-flaxseed oil 2 tbsp. Daily -calcium and seaweed for trace minerals

Hydrotherapy-avoid sunbathing face -fever treatment- the short cold bath

-full bath with warm clay baths (fill tub with thick clay paste at 102 degrees x 3-4 hours) warning-use tub outdoor -messy -hot foot bath –hot- 1 min/ tepid 30 sec-steam bath / salt bath 2x weekly

BLADDER

Causes:-trying to retain urine -kidney stones -bacteria invasion from poor health care-in men this is a signal of prostate problems-(_cyclamate_ -in artificial sugars causesbladder tumors)

Atony:-ascending jet or spray directly upward against the perineum, in addition a spray to the front of the abdomen only **-** Ascending Douche. This is a jet or spray directed upward, in this case, against the perineum). Abdominal Douche -a spray to the front of the abdomen only

Congested bladder Tea- 1 oz. Each couch grass, buchu, marshmallow+ 1 11/2 pints water- simmer for 15 min. 1cup q4h

-1oz, each horsetail grass+ shepherd's purse and bearberry leaves- 1-2 tsp. To 1 cup boil h20- cool and drink 1-2 cups daily

Insufficiency: spinal dorsal spray= hand held water hose to upper, and central part of spine- stream rapidly spray up and down spine extending 3-4 inches on either side of thespine (if spine origin- use tepid water) Give tepid water for irritability of the bladder (when of spinal origin). Give a Cold Spinal Douche for symptoms resulting in urinary incontinence or retention

Irritable bladder:-if no inflammation-hot sitz bath for 5 minutes followed by neutral sitz bath for 10- 20 minutes -hot pack to pelvis -heating compress over perineum and genitals - hot colonic. Revulsive Sitz,

Paresis(paralysis):-daily colonic -cold plantar spray to bottom of feet

Daily colonic. Cold Plantar Douche (that is, to bottom of feet) ; _sitz bath_

-uva-ursi, horse tail, buchu, chickweed, yerba manse, pipsissewa, burnet hydrangea, chaparral, devil's claw

Infection:-buchu tea 2 cups daily, cranberry 2 cups daily,

Cranactin- 3 capsules 2 x daily

-two day juice fast- carrot or citrus juice + 1 qt. Of either of the following *herbteas*: juniper (3 tbs. To 1 qt. Water) (soak juniper berries overnight) or corn silk (3 tbs.to 1 qt. Boiling water)- steep for 20 minutes and use as juice fast for 2 days

-*Garlic*-Drink tea made from 2-3 crushed or blended garlic bulbs several times a day.

-*Herbs*-Helpful herbs include juniper, lovage, parsley, uvaursi, rupturewort, bearberry, birch, and prickly restharrow.

-*Hydro*-A hot water bottle placed in direct contact to the urethral and vaginal openings may reduce pain. A heat lamp can also be used.

-*Juice*-Also drink cranberry juice. When you have this problem, citrus juice is not as good, since it tends to make the urine more alkaline, encouraging bacterial growth.

Bleeding:-golden seal- will stop it in 1 application and ½ tsp. Cayenne orally 3x daily

Inflammation—Copious water drinking; Revulsive Sitz Bath, twice a day; Hot Leg Packs followed by dry heat (Radiant Heat bath) to legs; Neutral Bath for 20-40 minutes, 2-3 times a week; prolonged Neutral Sitz Bath; Cold Mitten Friction; Cold Towel Rub; Fomentation over bladder; Hot Enema; Hot Pelvic Pack;

Hot water bottles ,heating pad brings relief place directly to the urethral and vaginal opening- hot sitz bath (105-115 f.) For 3-5 min. Or soak in tub- heat lamp

- do not apply- cold sitz bath, cold-full bath, cold douche

-hot enema

-use a Foley catheter and inject catnip tea in bladder

Retention: Lumbar Revulsive Douche. This spray should be hot, and then very brief cold, and will help alleviate urinary retention, due to spasm in the neck of the bladder

Stone gravel/ stones in the bladder: couch grass, gravel root

-Do not apply Cold Sitz Bath, Cold Full Bath, Cold Douche, or Cold Foot Bath.

Pain-To relieves the pain and encourages healing, take hot sitz (sitting) baths twice a day, for 20 minutes. To one of those daily sitz baths, add

1 cup of vinegar. The next day, add 2 cloves crushed garlic or garlic juice to the water of one of the two baths. **-**Supplement-Avoid zinc and iron supplements until this problem is healed.

Pain in the bladder on urination, with bloody urine, some gravel, and a slight fever of infection, proceed as follows:

3 parts goldenseal +2 parts gravel root+ 2 parts juniper berry+1 part buchu+1 part +marshmallow root

Use 1 part of shepherd's purse)= 10 parts total of active ingredients use 1 part slippery elm put all the herbs together and pulverize in a blender or mill then mix with enough liquid to make a dough-like consistency. For the liquid use a tincture of one of the herbs you have used, or use water. Mix a little liquid at a time to make the dough. Then roll the pills in your hand. Use about 1/8 teaspoon of the dough. Make the pills as large as the person can swallow. Put the pills on a cookie tray and bake at 200-250 degrees for 15-30 minutes to completely evaporate the water or alcohol. Give about six pills. Opt. Dip them one by one in olive oil / coconut oil and they will go down more easily. An infusion is a tea made by putting the herb (leaf, blossom, or stem) in a container and pouring hot water over it, and letting it set for 15-30 minutes. Roots and barks and seeds need simmer for 15 to 45 minutes to extract the properties.

Take-**a**=acute; **sa**=subacute; **c**=chronic; **d**=degenerative

-drink large quantities of water- 1/2 pint every 20 min. For 3 hours- then 1 cup every hour ,cranberry juice taken in place of a meal -chamomile, goldenseal, buchu, mint, and parsley tea(do not add sweetener or milk) -tea made from 2-3 cloves of crushed garlic- drink it several times per day	**A**-(cystitis) flaxseed, chaparral, cayenne, juniper berries **Sa**- (catarrh)white pond lily root, wild yam, goldenseal, capsicum, juniper berries **C**-(flaccidity) hyssop, parsley, juniper berries **D**-(degenerative stage) Echinacea, goldenseal, myrrh, chaparral

BLEED

General information <u>-all internal hemorrhage-saline enema retain when absorbed repeat</u> (1 tsp. Salt in 1 pt. Water 100-105F)	**Nose hemorrhage of the nose:** sniff goldenseal tea, ice to nose and back of neck, hot foot bath **Stomach bleeding-hemorrhage / ulcers:** -goldenseal

-hydrotherapy caution- do not use heat causes more bleeding-avoid cold full baths+ steam baths+ cold sprays *-herbal:* cayenne*, ginger -goldenseal internally and externally-plantain tea, hazelnut, burnet, smartweed, -mullein, grapevine, milfoil, horsetail, pauD'Arco, shepherd purse, selfheal, bilberry, comfrey root, turmeric, and bistort ,red raspberry leaves -nettle, comfrey, red root, yarrow -white oak bark+ witch hazel are especially good -*bayberry use alone or for better effect mix with *capsicum* *apply powder of bistort root to area*-blackberry *use short time (high tannin)-cramp bark*-dong quai* use for hemorrhage of all kinds, horsetail, Kentucky coffee- tree *-supplements:*-vitamin-c -vitamin -k (400mcg daily) -vitamin-e 800iu daily *-to prevent bleeding:* -vitamin-k 100mcg 3x daily **Bowel bleeding:**-keep pt. Lying, -warm herb enema-lie down-inject a tea of red raspberry tea, white oak bark or wild alum -2-3 oz. Retain as long as possible- then repeat also drink the tea -drink- shepherd's purse, raspberry leaves, bistort root, witch hazel, bayberry or sumac (use one or a mixture of 2-3)- drink 2 8 oz. Glasses daily **Chronic hemorrhage:** prepare an infusion of 1 tsp. Tormentil root powder into 1cups of hops infusion- drink 1 cups 4x daily- he recommends giving 2 fl.oz. Of tormentil tea every 1/2 hour	-swallow bits of ice rapidly for a short time and put ice over area -briefly apply ice over the stomach -witch hazel tea -red raspberry tea -bistort root-wild alum root -yarrow / sumac (steep a tsp. Of the herb in a cup of boiling water for 30 minutes strain and drink) -give a cupful of shepherd purse tea (a tea made of white oak bark or witch hazel is equally good) **Uterus hemorrhage:**-lay on back and elevate feet Give a hot douche of herbs (bayberry/ bistort) or one of above mentioned herbs) steep 1 tbs. Of herb in a qt. Of boiling water for 10 minutes (if herbs are granulated use 2 tbs. To 1 qt. Of boiling water- steep for 20 minutes- let stand strain and apply as hot as possible -hot douche of goldenseal tea -very cold water spray to the perineum -herbs-horseweed, smartweed ,infusion of powdered acorn or powdered cups **Wound bleeding womb and tumors:**-vitamin-k 400 mcg daily -vitamin-e 800 iu. Daily -peach leaf tea 4-5 cups daily -sarsaparilla 8-10 capsules daily -cayenne- 1tsp in 1 oz. Warm water drink 3x daily -shepherd purse 4 capsules daily -cold sitz baths -hot enema as needed for bleeding

until excessive discharge stops - prepare an infusion of hops tea- stir in 1 tsp. Tormentil root into 1 cup of thehops infusion - drink 1 cups 4x daily

Cut/ wound:-apply pressure, ice- apply cayenne powder to area

-slice grapefruit +salt and place on area

-dampen plantain/ marigold leaf and apply to wound

-witch hazel to area/ apply slum

-shepherd purse- drink and apply to area -mash juniper berries on bleeding wound

-very hot , very cold applications,

-squeezing lemon juice on the wound will immediately stop the wound-put citrus peeling powder to wound on the wound

Hemorrhoids bleeding: inject lemon juice in rectum

Lungs bleeding: very hot application to spine between shoulders -ice to chest-ice to hands-hot leg packs -elevate chest and shoulders -keep extremities warm

-cayenne-shepherd purse, goldenseal, plantaintea of white oak bark / witch hazel

-hot footbath + make a tea of cayenne and hemlock spruce

-cough as little as possible -swallow a pinch of cayenne(it will stop the bleeding almost immediately)

-a tea made from white oak bark or witch hazel

Reflex pressure area for hemorrhage-apply very cold-*32-40 degrees f. Or very hot (110-115 degrees f.) For.......*

-*brain*- apply to face, scalp, back of neck, hands, feet, legs

-*heart*-area above heart

-*intestine*-entire abdomen

-*kidneys + intestines* - lower dorsal and lumbar spine

-*kidneys and ureters*- central abdomen- from navel to pubis

-*liver* skin over lower right chest walls

-*lungs*-chest (front and back), dorsal region, shoulders, feet, legs

-*nose*-mucous membrane, hands- (hot nasal spray)- ice collar

-*pharynx and larynx*- neck

-*spleen*- skin over left chest walls

-*pelvic organs*(uterus, ovaries, bladder, rectum) -lower lumbar and sacral spine, lower abdomen, groin and upper inner surface of thigh, feet, legs, breast

Prostate and seminal vesicles- inner thigh

-*stomach*-epigastric region

-*vagina*-hot vaginal douche

hemorrhage excessive: -smartweed -burnet –hazelnut

-tormentil tea as an infusion- every 1/2 hour until bleeding stops-.herbs: -persimmon bark tea* -bilberry -comfrey root -white oak bark

BLOOD	
Cholesterol, Circulation &/or Blood Pressure Tincture: -Use the above Cayenne Pepper Tincture Method with 3 parts - Red Clover Blossoms, 2 parts - Garlic, 1 part - Ginger Root and 1 part - Cayenne Pepper. -Take 2-3 Dropperfuls - 3-4 times per Day, if needed. **Need vitamin**-b12, for formation of blood cells- vitamin-c	**Chlorophyll cocktail=**red blood cell builder *wheat grass For blood 4 beet tops- handful of parsley- handful of spinach-6 carrots -½ tomatoes **Formula blood building:** alfalfa 1 oz. + parsley root 1oz. + ½ oz. Each of (dandelion, burdock, comfrey, Yellow dock, nettles, dulse)- simmer in 1 qt. Water in covered pot, cool, strain-return liquid

Purifying and sweating tea- ½ oz. Elder + ½ oz. Peppermint in 1 pt. Water

Supplement-clay + Swedish bitters- blood purifier, blood vessel health- silicon damaged blood vessels- boswelia

Blood cleanser: red clover and paud'arco chaparral, Echinacea, red- clover, burdock, myrrh, Oregon grape root, pauD'Arco, dandelion, yellow dock ,*holy thistle *sassafras, chicory*culver's root*alfalfa*devil's claw* watercress*yucca herb

-formula: 1 cup of red clover + 1 cup burdock + 4 tbs. Yellow dock mix in 2 qt. Of water make tea - drink 1 qtr. Daily

Blood thinner: garlic

to pot, simmer uncovered for 1 hour until it is reduced to 1 cup-stir in 1 cup of unsulfured blackstrap molasses- refrigerate- take 1 tbs. 3xdaily or #00 capsules 2-4 with each meal

Blood poisoning: -symptom- rapid pulse, chills, red around the wound-take a high enema, fruit juices , echenesia

Blood vessels- take silicon supplement, vanadium (arteries)gingko- strengthens blood vessels

Blood clotting prevention: angelica, anise, fenugreek, garlic, ginger, ginkgo, ginseng, meadowsweet, motherwort, myrrh, and turmeric.

Horse chestnut seed to prevent clots

BLOOD POISON-Emergency room= fatal

Symptoms:- severe localized pain and discoloration, swelling, red streaks from the wound which extend up the veins toward the heart. High fever, chills, violent shivering, pale, restless, irritable, sores which do not heal.

Apply -If discharge from the wound is thin, apply powdered 50-50 myrrh and goldenseal directly to the wound.

-poultice of lemons or charcoal. Or crush one or more of the herbs listed later in this article.

Drink tea: chickweed, plantain, goldenseal and myrrh chickweed, and myrrh.

Cups of Echinacea tea a day as possible. -Echinacea tea,-Drink charcoal water

Formula: -4 tbs. Each yellow dock, 4 tbsp. Red clover, burdock root, and 1 tbsp. Blood root,-put them in 1 1/2 qt. Boil. Water- simmer reduce to 1 qt. -strain, add honey, and1 pt. Glycerin- mix-keep cool -take- 2 fl.oz. 3-4 x daily

Take a high enema + fast

Hydro-hot fomentations- two of them to effected area then place a cold towel over the area -alternating hot and cold -40°c degrees (104°f degrees) for 2 minutes +cold 30 sec., repeat 2X . Until the red lines disappear

Poultice: lemon/ charcoal to area

Wound: wash area with boric acid

Chilly: give cayenne water

BONE

Note:-calcium is essential ,when certain minerals aremissing in the diet- calcium is reabsorbed out of the bones (causing bones to behoneycomb-porous- easily break)

-calcium-phosphorus imbalances caused by too much phosphorus in the diet-lack of exercise and other hormones causes bone problems

-lack of hydrochloric acids in the stomach causes poor calcium absorption(HCL is needed for calcium and other mineral absorption)

Check vitamin-c deficiency

Calcium formula: comfrey root 4 tbs. + horsetail grass 6 tbsp.+ oat straw 3 tbs. Lobelia 1 tbs. Nettles 3 tbs. This is an excellent calcium formula to rebuild weak bones- take 4cups 3x daily (this also relieves pain-calcium smoothie- ¼ bunch parsley +1 cup pineapple juice- blend till smooth. Drink

Old folks remedy that works-boil water and place olive oil in glass jar to heat up in boiled water and rub on area -will speed up healing

Supplement- see skeletal system

Possible causes of bone disease:- avoid excess calcium supplements when confined to bed during healing(causes stones) -vinegar and meat decreases bone mass-caffeine, alcohol refined sugars are all harmful to the bones-excess fat intake decreases bone mass -cola drink causes calcium loss(a tooth place in cola drink will disappear in an hour)

-avoid chard, spinach, rhubarb, poke (high oxalic acid causes bone loss)

-those with bone disease should limit eating(tomatoes, eggplant, bell peppers, \white potatoes with green to skin)- they contain the calcium inhibitor

Horsetail extract is a good source of silica

BONE SPUR-derived colloidal minerals tend to reverse spurs and calcium deposits, without surgery, by remodeling the bones

-*pain* -bromelain and turmeric -1-2 weeks fast and cleanse -only drink distilled water -hot-cold foot baths -walk barefoot outside -stretching exercises

Give vitamin C to bowel tolerance, along with vitamin E and

Magnesium. Correct the calcium/phosphorous ratio by taking 2,000 mg of calcium a day.

BOWEL

Chlorophyll heals-fast 1-2 days per week, bowel tissue damage, rebuilds the tissues

Bowel inflammation/ dysentery

Charcoal water (drink + put poultice over stomach andbowels) and put charcoal poultice over the stomach

Gas fermentation*anise

Bowel fever- *bistort root*

Disinfect- chlorophyll

Bowel pain- common evening primrose

BRAIN

Brain Tincture:

Use the above Cayenne Pepper Tincture Method with 3 parts - Ginkgo Biloba Leaf, 1 part

Take 2-3 Dropperfuls - 3-4 times per Day, if needed. - Rosemary Leaf, 1 part Kola Nut and 1 part - Cayenne Pepper.

BREAST

Herbs-a=acute; **sa**=subacute; **c**=chronic; **d**=degenerative

A-(mastitis) comfrey, goldenseal, slippery elm

Sa-(congestion, engorgement) sanicle, black cohosh, chaparral

C-(cyst) castor bean, Echinacea, burdock, chaparral

D- (degenerative stage) chaparral, Echinacea, goldenseal, greater celandine

For breast tenderness- take selenium-apply vitamin E on the area, and be sure to include enough essential fatty acids in the diet (5 gm, 3 times a day). Flaxseed oil, sunflower seed oil, or wheat germ oil are best.

Breast cyst -_Apply-_ primrose oil will help reduce the cysts.

Hydrotherapy some find that applying cold water to the breasts helps when they are painful; or alternating very warm and cold. This can be done via heating pads, cold cloths, showers, etc.

_Take-_the trace element, germanium, is important. It is found in garlic and onions.

Benign breast changes:-Regularly take B vitamins, vitamin C, calcium, and magnesium. . Do not use diuretic drugs. Instead, drink more water to help improve kidney function. Do not use highly salted foods.

-Dong quai helps regulate hormonal levels.

Breast inflammation -Soak a cloth in a mixture of 1 pint of linseed oil and 4 ounces of spirits of camphor, and cover the entire affected area. Apply as often as needed. -Hot and cold applications of dry cloths help relieve the soreness and inflammation. Give these continually until relieved. Then reapply the mixture - poultice slippery elm, with a little lobelia added to it. -Drink a tea of goldenseal, black cohosh, and ginger.	-Goldenseal helps heal infections. Red clover cleans the blood. -Chlorophyll - clean the liver and prevent formation of cysts. -Germanium and coq10 -Flaxseed oil helps prevent breast cancer.
BRONCHITIS	
Cause:-infections by chemicals or physical agents such as fumes, smoke (chief cause) ,dust, etc. -children in homes where gas is used for cooking have a higher incident than those where electric stove is used-study shows milk as a cause -*often caused by constipation* **Symptoms:-**generally begins with an upper respiratory infection, gradual unset of cough, mucous -wheezing and acute respiratory distress follows-may be fever, chilliness, muscle aches, headaches, hoarseness, and dryscratchy throat -chronic bronchitis- caused by repeated bouts of acute Bronchitis from allergies, irritants etc. **Cough** 1x per minutes for 20 minutes **Cayenne and lobelia** will help break up the congestion. **Herbs-**catnip, comfrey, goldenseal, mullein, yarrow, myrrh, pau D'Arcy, chickweed, gingko bilboa, burdock, lobelia, slippery elm bark ,wild cherry bark , Echinacea, cayenne, garlic, Venus maidenhair fern- used as an expectorant - *grape seed extract Calamint , *chamomile, * elecampane, eucalyptus, hore hound, lung wort, pleurisy root , *licorice -marshmallow, *common catalpa -*Irish moss, lemon balm **Formula: see respiratory therapy** 1 cups of honey + 1/3tsp ginger + 1/3 tsp cayenne	**Lemon** water 6-8 glasses daily- **Anise tea and almond** milk are helpful in bronchitis. Make the almond milk by blending 6 tbsp. Of almonds in a pint of water. **Supplements:** -vitamin-c to bowel tolerance -vitamin b6 200 mcg daily **A hot footbath** will help pull the blood away from the chest and reduce congestion **Steam Epson salt** bath for 15 minutes (2lbs.) **Apply warm, moist heat or** a hot water bottle over the chest and back before bedtime. This will help relieve congestion and aid in sleep - hot foot bath with 1 tbsp. Mustard- heating compress at night cover with plastic bag and sweater **Take enough** water intake **Vaporizer** with eucalyptus or peppermint oil breath for 10-15minutes- 3-4x/D **Deep breathing exercises** hold for a few seconds 10-20x **Cough:-** heating chest pack - irritable cough without expectoration- gargle hotwater-warm vapor inhalation- cough with copious expectoration-copious hot water drinking, fomentation to chestevery 2 hours **Painful cough- fomentation** to chest every 2 hours Dry cotton chest pack

-lobelia tincture (excellent bronchodilator)

-garlic-mix thyme powder with honey- take 1 spoonful as needed-1 tsp. Thyme leaves + 1 cup boiling water- pour over herb and cover. Steep for 20 minutes- strain and drink 3 cups daily

-anise tea + almond milk- blend 6 tbs. Of almonds in 1 pt. Of water to make almond milk (reported helpful)

-mullein 8 oz. In tea pot inhale the steam -mullein 8 oz. And fenugreek tea (1 tsp. Per cup) for several weeks

-1 cup honey +1/3 tsp. Ginger + 1/3 tsp. Cayenne

-non-productive cough- percussion to chest

Hot and cold treatments to chest 3 minutes hot 30 seconds cold

Congestion: -swallow a little *cayenne* and lobelia

Irritable cough, without*expectoration*—Sip very hot water; gargle hot water; Steam Inhalations; avoid mouth breathing; keep air of room warm (75^0-80^0F.) And moist with -take an emetic- add 1/2 tsp lobelia to 1 qt. Boiled water -let steep when warm drink as much as possible -run finger down throat till vomit then take a high enema

BURN

1ˢᵗ apply cool water to stop the burn use in even 3ʳᵈ degree burns

Formula burn- honey +olive

Oil/ 2tbs. Comfrey + 1 tbsp. Wheat germ oil + 1 tbs.

Honey poultice- mix with olive oil and apply it prevents shock, scarring, pneumonia (1 part olive oil to 2 part honey) -or aloe Vera -apply vitamin-e/ a -apply fresh comfrey/ clary/ baking soda paste

-Fresh aloe Vera juice

Apply-*mashed onions- olive* oil- *castor* oil- *baking soda* diluted make paste sesame seed oil, *coconut* oil,

-grated raw potatoes-sweet almond oil

-alternate with olive oil and aloe at night

-vitamin -e oil or vitamin an oil*

-lavender oil 25 drops+ 2 oz. Distilled water + and witch hazel, store in refrigerator—use spray bottle excellent

-paste of wheat germ oil + honey in blender on low speed --then add comfrey leaves to make a thick

Paste (keep refrigerated)- cold clay poultice- day and night

Excessive burns: continuous neutral full bath till healed

Old burns: paraffin bath -burns take 3-6 months to heal -.apply aloe

Electrical:-call 911 -do not touch victim -turn off power source if possible

-if unconscious -check for CPR need -use wood to push power away from victim

-do not cool the burn area -do not move him except for CPR (may have spinal injury)-keep from getting chill-look for 2 wounds (entrance and exit site of power)

Grease burn:-do not add anything but cold water-do not remove blister from skin-do not pull clothing of the skin -keep bandage loose-do not put honey, butter or vegetable peeling on (it will seal the heat in)-with finger remove burn area off skin (this will allow blood to area)

Hot tar / wax: -use ice water to harden and remove-after it is remove use no more ice ,but cool water

Sun burn:-oatmeal water compress -aloe -t-tree -clay poultice -witch hazel -plain yogurt to area -cucumber -raw eggplant -plantain -soda alkaline bath

-apply compress of this solution 15-20 minutes daily

-in Russia raw eggs smeared over area and washed off after 20 minutes with amazing results

Painful burns:-apply vitamin-e and spray a 3% solution of vitamin-c to area every 2-4 hours-take 1000mg vitamin -c every hour -ice water compress

Large burns : -blend aloe leaves with a tiny drop of lemon apply if no aloe - apply cold water **Acid burn:** -baking soda, or apple cider added to warm water- do it 5 minutes daily **Chemical:-**flush area with cool water -remove clothes if with chemical	
BURSITIS	
=**inflammation of the liquid-**filled sac joint **Swedish bitters**- use as compress to area +/ **DMSO** **Vitamin E**, protein and vitamins A and C increases during infection. Vitamin B_{12} is also helpful. Flaxseed oil **Herbs:-**ginger combine with pineapple and licorice-*devil's claw	**During the initial phase-** apply ice pack (ice massage) for 30 min. Every 2-3 hours-hip area sit in cold water in tub -as pain decreases hot fomentation-start ones pain decrease for 45-60 min.- follow with range of motion exercises -**Hot castor oil** packs are useful

CANCER

SYMPTOMS

Bladder and Kidney: Blood in urine and increased urination frequency. Bloody urine is possibly cancer

Breast: Lump which is hard, does not go away, and does not move; inflammation or thickening of the skin.

Cervical and Uterine: Bleeding between periods, unusual discharge, painful periods, and heavy periods.

Colon: Blood in stools, rectal bleeding, changes in bowel habits (diarrhea and/or *constipation*).

Endometrium: Bleeding between menstrual periods, unusual discharge, painful periods, and heavy periods.

Skin cancer: A lump under the skin, moles which change color or size and have raised edges, an ulcer which does not heal, flat sores, lesions which like moles.

Larynx: Persistent cough and hoarse throat.

Lung: Persistent cough, bloody sputum, and chest pain.

Leukemia: Whiteness of skin, weight loss, fatigue, repeated infections, easy bruising, nosebleeds.

Lymphoid Tissue: Enlarged, rubbery, lymph nodes; itching; night sweats; unexplained fever and/or weight loss.

Mouth or throat: Chronic ulcer of the mouth, tongue, or throat which not heal.

Ovaries: Usually there are no obvious symptoms until later stages.

Prostate: Weak or interrupted urine flow; continuous pain in lower back, pelvis, +/or upper thighs.

Stomach: Indigestion and pain after eating.

Testicles: Enlargement of a testicle, thickening of scrotum, lumps, sudden excess of fluid in scrotum, mild ache in lower abdomen or groin.

Avoid salt- iron supplement encourages cancer growth, cured, smoked, or nitrite-cured foods. Alcohol- linked to cancer

Herbs: pau D'Arcy, ginseng, licorice, esiac tea, citrus pectin, -Ojibwa herbal tea=burdock, slippery elm, sheep sorrel and turkey rhubarb-olive leaf extract, gingko, cat's claw, chlorella, coumarin, Echinacea extract, garlic, pau D'Arcy, mistletoe, ginseng, seaweed extract, shiitake mushroom, turmeric

Tea as an enema- 1/2 oz. To 1 pint of water-inject in morning and night

-intestinal cleanser-use it about three times a day, At the same time do a retention enema to replenish the acidophilus (one tbs. +plus one tablespoon whey, mix that in about 8 ounces warm water. And slowly inject that into the colon)

Cleanser: oral cleanser- 3x daily -coffee enema- 3tbs ground (not instant) to 1 qt. Waterlet boil x 3 minutes and simmer x 15 minutes-**raw food only-** ginger, carrots, cleanse,(juicing), barley green

Juice daily: not canned-orange, carrot, green leaf, grape, grapefruit, apple **treatment diet plan**

*Day 1-2 fast-*repeat fast 1-2 days weekly

Day 2- take 16 oz. Fresh grape juice 3x daily may dilute

Day-3- switch to 16 oz. Fresh carrot juice 3x daily

Day-4- use grape juice at dinner and carrot juice at breakfast

Day-5- 10 -use the same juices- in addition to grape juice eat any kind of raw fruit and in addition to carrot juice eat any type of raw vegetables

Day 11-15 :begin adding stewed and steamed vegetables serve hot, no salt- never overeat -toxins

Day 16- begin taking 3 almonds with breakfast and dinner- small fruits for dinner as soon as you can go to 2 meal plan

Day-17- add 1/2 cup brown rice

*Day 18-20-*increase quantity of rice by 1/4 per day till reach 1 cup serve with fruits, onions, tomatoes lemon juice, or green peas -no seasons

If had chemo- do 2-3 coffee enemas daily -do 5 coffee enemas daily

Green leaf juice: use any of the above as many combined as you can find-lettuce, Swiss chard, escarole, romaine, watercress, greens(turnip, collard, mustard) red cabbage 2-3 leaves, beet tops as young inner leaves green pepper 1/4 of small one, sprouts- (grind 2x)-press and drink immediately

Excellent-papaya seed, avocado seed, papaya leaf, corosol, , barley green

-laetrile (b17)containing foods (ginger , apricot/ almond/ peach / apple seed, tamarind)

Eat raw, eat a little seaweed daily

-eat tomatoes- contains lycopene an antioxidant

-broccoli and dark green leafy vegetables fights cancer- broccoli, Brussels sprouts, and cauliflower contains d-glutamic acid which reduces various cancers

-cherries especially tart ones- prevent cancer

-the only added sweetener should be a little honey/ blackstrap molasses'

-soybeans contains genistein and diadzein - antioxidants

-high dose of vitamin-C

-*citrus pectin*- inhibit the metastatic spread of cancer by 80%

-*Chaparral*,paud'arco-excellent- wheat grass juice, esiac tea

-drink *red clover* tea all day like water

-fast+ carrot juice fast has been proven

-*asparagus and garlic* (anti-cancer)

Strain-chamomile tea enema- 1 cup flower to 1 pt. Water simmer x 30 minutes incovered saucepan.- strain can keep in glass--dish no longer than 3 days

Formula: red clover 4part, burdock 4 part, yellow dock 3 part, blue violet 3partgoldenseal 1 part, myrrh 1/2 part, Echinacea 3 part, aloes 1 part, blue flag 1 part, gravel root 2 part, blood root 2 part, dandelion 2 part African cayenne 1 part, chickweed 2 part, Oregon grape 2 parts

Day 21- increase number of high protein foods served(eat 85- 95% raw)-asparagus and garlic = anti-cancer *no sugar, salt, baking powder or baking soda-*

Use peppermint tea when unable to tolerate food 1 tbsp. To 8 cups water boil x - 5 minutes strain

Crush raw garlic let it set out in room temperature open air or 10 minutes is powerful blend in v-8 and drink

Only drink distilled water-

Avoid- animal products of all kinds including milk -do not use aluminum utensils

Sunshine- daily exercise-if too week ,do massage daily x 10 days than 2x weekly-distilled water only 8- 14

Hydrotherapy:-fever bath- 102-105 degrees x 5-15 minutes 5x weekly 2-4 x weeks or 2x weeklyfor months-do salt glow -daily skin brushing - see Russian steam

Castor oil pack to area

Skin -*formula*:= parts: bees wax, resin, vegetable fat, garlic poultice, sheep poulticesheep sorrel (heat x 20 minutes cool with 1/2 to 1 cup of olive oil whip and cool-wear at night under bandage) -five lb. Young poke raw make a paste. Mix 1 lb. Blood root 3lb. Raw garlic (make paste and mix all together and apply as needed for 8-10 days)

In Australia they use:--raw eggplant to skin and ginseng extracts

Malignant sores:- fig poultice-*carrot poultice- *cleavers, chaparral-*use sorrel to cure skin cancer

Liver and pancreatic cancer-Supplements:-green foods. Flax-oil 2 tsp daily, milk thistle seed, shiitake mushroom**,** dandelion, ginkgo , paud'arco, Echinacea, goldenseal, saw palmett,Ginseng/ licorice elixir, coq-10 300mg daily, l-carnitine 500mg daily, chromium picolate 250 mcg daily, glutathione 100mg daily-vitamin-c 10,000 with bioflavonoids daily

Vaginal: blended raw garlic douche

-liver building juice: 6 lemon + 1cup molasses, 2 tbsp. Beet powder,1/2 tsp cayenne,4 tbsp. Alfalfa, 12 oz. Water-mix together-	

CANDIDA

Symptoms:-*both sexes* have itching in genital area, discomfort during urination, *Women-* thick ,odorless vaginal discharge-this is not a venereal disease but a yeast infection that can be transmitted by sexual contact and other ways Bad breath, constipation, chronic yeast infections, depression, fatigue, food cravings, gas, persistent bloating, headache, brain fog, adrenal and thyroid problems, vaginal(white itchy cheese-like) infections, hiatal hernia, insomnia, mental confusion,-simple test to see if you have candida **Normal candida diet:** no sugar or other sweeteners. No canned or dried fruit or fruit juice of any kind. Very limited less sweet fruits, such as a raw apple two or three times a week. <u>No yeast</u> breads or yeast flakes. No foods containing vinegar, such as mayonnaise or pickles. No fermented foods, such as soy sauce. No fruit of any kind should be eaten. Abundance of vegetables, legumes, and a modest amount of whole grains such as barley and oatmeal waffles for a bread substitute and brown rice. Nuts and seeds, except peanuts, are acceptable in the diet if they are free from all molds. Avocadoes and olives, along with nuts	**Test-** 1st thing in morning, spit in a glass of water, wait for 1 hour if a cloud is on bottom of glass or string like material floating on top you have candida, if nothing happens you don't have candida **Herbs:** burdock, Echinacea, ginger, goldenseal, bee pollen, kelp, lobelia, passion flower,*paud'arco, psyllium, slippery elm, ginkgo, suma **Supplements:** liquid kyolic garlic: 1 teaspoon, 3x a day, for one month, then kyolic reserve capsules (the strongest garlic capsules available), 1 capsule, 3x a day, to be continued as long as the *candida* persists. -goldenseal herb: ¼ teaspoon powder, 2x a day. -uvaursi herb: ¼ teaspoon powder, 2x a day. -probiotics: take 2 tablets first thing in the morning and 2 tablets mid-afternoon. -olive leaf extract is an antifungal agent, and might be worth trying. **Grape seed extract-excellent** **30-day grapefruit seed extract "cure"** use 8-16 drops in each quart of water taken.

CATARACT

Symptom:-lenses of the eye becomes clouded **Lemon drop** in morning and drop of honey at night x 30 days **Enema** 2x daily for 7 days only1-2 qtr. Carrot juice daily -take juice of 3 lemons in 1 pt. Water every morning- 1 hour before breakfast **Eyebright** 2x daily(1/2tsp./ glass of water) 3 cups bilberry tea daily (1 tbsp. Of herb per cup of water)	**Vitamins-** see daily recommended dose below –D(600 iu.) Daily A(50,000 iu). Daily- E (600)-C- 5000 mg 2x daily-B12- 50- B-2 – 50 mg daily--riboflavin 1000mg daily-B complex 300mg **Hot / cold compress** to eye, hot salt water fomentations over closed eye **inflammation -** (charcoal and flaxseed/ slippery elm poultice)-daily- apply cold to the eye; white of an egg on paper towel over the eye

Herbs: rinse eye with eye cup using = part eyebright, goldenseal, bayberry 3xdaily- and take orally teas from these herbs - 1 1/2 qtr. Of carrot juice daily	**Red raspberry, cayenne** -acidophilus 3 cap 3x daily-wash eyes with infusion of **Swedish bitters**- compress to closed eyes for 1 hour daily

CELIAC (Gluten Intolerance)

Symptom; symptoms usually begins under 1 year of age -occasionally cases begins in teens or adults -excess gas, diarrhea (most common symptom) - weight loss- wasting -stunt growth- stool-bulky, pale , light, yellow, foul, floats -abdomen swelling- may develop blisters or sores all over their body irritability, behavioral changes-(the disease can begin in the first few months of life) **Cause:-**it is a disease of the small intestines-abnormality in the intestinal lining due to permanent intolerance to gluten-gluten intolerance= wheat, rye , barley, oats-cow milk allergies - sometime develop before the celiac symptoms Avoid the gluten foods, which are wheat, oats, rye, and barley. The follow grains do not have gluten: corn, millet, and rice. Quince, soybeans, and amaranth are also okay. Buckwheat is okay for some celiac, but not for others.	**Ripe bananas-**aids in the control ofdiarrhea, acidophilus **Supplements:** check for anemia , vitamin -a, k, d, b12, glutamine (500-1000 mg)- take for 1 year or more **Herbs:** burdock, aloe Vera, paud'arco, psyllium, saffron, slippery elm, alfalfa, garlic raw or cooked Helpful herbs include aloe Vera, burdock. **All grains fed to babies** (and adults too) should be cooked for 2-3 hours, Ripe bananas are tolerated well, and help control the diarrhea **Do not overeat sugar or white-**flour products -total healing may take 6 months to 1 year-occasionally may have to be treated for iron deficiency-*breast feed* to avoid the use of cow's milk-use rice, millet and corn instead of the gluten foods **Garlic(**contains allisatin)-reports to help,

CHLAMYDIA

Symptoms:-*women-* burning sensation when urinating, itching, painful intercourse, whitevaginal discharge (like cottage cheese)-*men-*often there is no symptoms, possible clear, watery urethral discharge **Bathe sores** 2-3 x daily with solution of goldenseal and myrrh	**Use vaginal suppository** of -t-tree oil nightly, hot foot bath with pinch of cayenne **Mix = part-** powdered goldenseal, barberry, oregano grape root with vit-a oil - soak in a cotton ball -insert as a tampon against the cervix

CHOLESTEROL
	Only found in animal products
Check copper deficiency **Cholesterol, Circulation &/or Blood** *Pressure Tincture:* -Use the above Cayenne Pepper Tincture Method with 3 parts - Red Clover Blossoms, 2 parts - Garlic, 1 part - Ginger Root and 1 part - Cayenne Pepper. -Take 2-3 Dropperfuls - 3-4 times per Day, if needed.	**Activated charcoal-**one quarter ounce (approximately one tablespoon) of activated charcoal three times daily **Daily sunshine** **Soybean (tofu),** red grape juice, grapefruit, tomato, apple, eggplant, corn, cabbage, peas, beans, green leafy vegetables, high fiber cereals **Brown rice diet** (rice and fruits only)- for 2-3 days decreases triglyceride (one person went from 1000 to 117 mg/dl)-drink 8 glasses of water daily

Sunshine-10-20 minutes daily exposure to sunshine decreases blood cholesterol

Supplements-vitamin-b15 (30mg daily) -copper (1-2 mg daily) -lecithin 1 tbsp. 2x daily-iodine -l-arginine 500mg/ (oat bran) - beet juice -grapefruit , oranges-flax meal- flax oil (vitamin-f) decreases chop. -rice yeast extract-vitamin-c (1000-400mg), niacin, vitamin-b5 pantothenic acid -niacin (1500mg daily) **:-** inositol

Carnitine- decreases triglyceride -beta-sitosterol-inhibit cholesterol in the blood

Vitamins C, E, b-complex and niacin also lower cholesterol, along with calcium

Kyolic may also lower cholesterol

- to keep cholesterol absorbing fiber flowing

Eat avocados, oat bran, garlic, onions, celery juice -they tend to lower cholesterol levels -prunes help reduce cholesterol

-amaranth ,lecithin, alfalfa meals, garlic-900mg daily, brewer's yeast, and chromium, flaxseed oil, Barley, spirulina, lemongrass oil, and activated charcoal.

Cut an eggplant and place in refrigerator in distilled water over-night- drink 3 cups daily

Oat bran lowers cholesterol

Psyllium seed also lowers it

CHROHN'S

Description - inflammation of the digestive tract it is similar to ulcerative colitis=autoimmune disease- toxic colon leading the body to get confused

Symptoms: diarrhea-4-5 stool daily and pain -fever, weight loss-abdominal masses may also be present -abdominal pain worsen with eating and improve with fasting -may have right lower quadrant pain-leading to pale, bulky stool that floats

Cabbage juice - *a fat-free diet*

Nutritional:-acidophilus (non-dairy)

-1 tsp three times daily -aloe vera drink -1/2 cup 2-3 cupsdaily-they do not tolerate fats (need a fat free diet) -avoid gas forming foods-avoid condiments-(peppers, mustard, horseradish, vinegar)-eliminate all food additives- (they irritate the bowels)-study shows improvement when placed on a sugar free diet- study shows gluten free diet beneficial: avoid gluten (found in wheat, oats, barley, rye, buckwheat)-avoid stress, worry, competitive games, anxiety- study shows(fiber-rich, unrefined carbohydrate diet-beneficial)-lactose intolerance is common-avoid overeating-cabbage juice

Diet-cabbage juice, olives, flaxseed and flaxseed oil (1-3 teaspoons, 1-3 times daily), celery (3 stalks pureed once or twice a day), nightshade free for 3 months trial (tomatoes, potatoes,

Avoid- stress, spicy food, greasy food, caffeine, alcohol, dairy products, eggs, carbonated drinks, etc. Start on a vegan diet avoid gluten (wheat, oat, rye, barley, buckwheat) -raw fruits and vegetables-never fry food

Vitamins: a lack of vitamin-c and e in the diet aggravates the problem-b-complex- 100mg 3x daily -b12 - 1000mcg daily -multivitamin- as directed-vitamin- e 800-1200iu daily -vitamin-a 25,000 iu. 2x daily-b-1 vitamin-glutamine (500-1000 mg)- take for 1 year or more if you have celiac, colitis, chromes

Herbs:-clay, echinacea 4 capsules 3x daily -paud'arcy - 4 capsules 3x daily -yerba mate - 3capsuls 3x daily-black walnut, burdock, goldenseal, psyllium ,saffron, aloe vera, fenugreek, \valerian, slippery elm, white oak bark, boswelia, turmeric-charcoal- helps control diarrhea-4-6 tabs 2-3x daily between meals

Formula:(move bowels daily)- mix one lb. Psyllium, 1/2 lb. Slippery elm, 4 tbsp. Chia seed(ground up), 1/2 cup of whey, mix all together -take 1 tbs. Of herb mix with 3 oz. Soy milk

Hydrotherapy:-daily warm bath (add 1/2 cup of ginger to water)-vapor steam bath daily- add 1tsp eucalyptus oil to vaporizer water under the chair- take hot bath and add 1 tsp eucalyptus to water take nightly.-daily warm baths add ½ cup ginger to water

eggplant, peppers, pimento, paprika), and gluten grains omitted (wheat, rye, barley, oats). Pineapple suppresses inflammation; so do apples and hawthorn berry tea.	**Diarrhea:-**charcoal- charcoal water or 4-6 tablets 2-3 times daily between meals

CIRCULATION POOR

Cholesterol, Circulation &/or Blood Pressure Tincture: -Use the above Cayenne Pepper Tincture Method with 3 parts - Red Clover Blossoms, 2 parts - Garlic, 1 part - Ginger Root and 1 part - Cayenne Pepper. -Take 2-3 Dropperfuls - 3-4 times per Day, if needed. **Emergency:** *drink cayenne water* swallow a little cayenne and water (goldenseal is also helpful)- *Take-***a**=acute; **sa**=subacute; **c**=chronic; **d**=degenerative **A**-(hemorrhage) wild alum root, bistort, goldenseal, sanicle **Sa**- (poor circulation) cayenne, ginger, prickly ash, goldenseal **C**-(varicose vein) wild alum root, goldenseal, St. John's wort, witch hazel **D**-(arteriosclerosis) fennel seed, fenugreek seed, Hawthorne berries, kelp **Swedish bitters**- improves circulation **Treatment:** cleanse, enema:- red raspberry tea enema 2x daily -high enemas, **Formula:-** take 1 part each cayenne, skullcap, and 1/2 part Goldenseal -garlic 1part, onion 1 part, ginger root 1/2 part(mix together in 4 parts water , drink 6oz. Daily) -1 part each- cayenne, goldenseal, skullcap+ 1/2 part goldenseal -1 tbsp. Yellow mustard powder,2 tbsp. Ginger powder + 1 tbsp. Cayenne	**Formula-**valerian- 2 part -spearmint 2 part -skullcap 2 part -gentian root 1 part-rue 2 part -catnip 1/2 part -cayenne pepper 1 part(mix use 1 tbsp. To 6 oz. Water to a tea 2x daily) **Take cool morning showers** or alternating hot and cold showers for 5 minutes morning and evening. Exercise afterward and make sure you are warm improve-alternate hot and cold to spine-local alternate bath (contrast baths)-painful sluggish circulation- see local alternate bath add 1/4 cup mustardpowder to water or 1 tsp cayenne Avoid hot tub bath -daily skin brushing *<u>do not do</u> hot and cold alt. Shower Early morning-cold shower / cool bath/ cold towel rub-Epson salt bath daily- use 4 lb. Per tub Head(to improve circulation of) -alternate hot and cold to head -deep breathing-cold mitten friction,/ cold shower in morning/ cool bath followed by rubbing with coarse towel **Herbs:** gingko, cinnamon and clove, gentian, coriander seed - bitter orange **Drink plenty ofred clover tea-cayenne pepper** 1 capsule 3x daily **Supplement:** niacin 50 mg 3x daily, folic acid, vitamin-e Take 800-1,200 IU of vitamin E daily. Take vitamin C to bowel tolerance. Also needed: niacin, RNA, and folic acid.

COLDSORES

Cause:- -stress -sugar and foods; herpes virus-occurs where the skin and mucus membranes meet(lining of eye lid, borders of mouth, gums)	**As soon as the first tingle is felt**, take 500 mg of Vitamin C with bioflavonoids, 3 times a day, for 3 days.

-last 7-10 days -usually reoccur in same spot **1st sign** apply ice to area for 15-20 minutes	**Vitamin**-b complex, e, a , lysine **herbs: -**gold-enseal, Echinacea, red clover, pau d'arco, black walnut tincture

COLDS /FLU

See gastroenteritis (stomach flu) **Caution**-legionnaire's, see meningitis- stiff neck-see mononucleosis- swollen glands, jaundice, red rash-see toxic shock-sore throat, sudden vomit, confusion, diarrhea See mononucleosis-flu last 2-4 weeks **Cut a clove** of garlic and put in ear **1st sigh:- enema** at First symptom **Formula-**1/2 tsp. Peppermint oil+ 1 cup honey+ 1/3 ginger + lemonjuice -simmer 1 tbs. Black walnut for 30 minutes in 1 qt. Water strain and drink theqt. Over the day **Blend-**6 lemons juiced, 2tsp ground ginger, 6-8 garlic cloves1/16 tsp cayenne, 4 cups water, 1/2-1 tsp honey to taste (opt.) **Russian penicillin**-wash 2 grapefruits and peel(cut peelings up thin.) Put peelings in Pot with 1 garlic bulb + 1 onions--add enough water to boil till garlic is tender-add a pinch of cayenne and-a handful of peach leaf or yarrow tea -mix add 1 ½qt. Water - drink 3 oz. Every hour till healed **Herbs-**elderberry extract-tincture goldenseal/ echenesia in throat, garlic, fast, cat's claw, pau d'arco **Hydrotherapy-**cold mitten friction, hot tub bath-add 2 cups of mustard powder to wateror add charcoal - bath additives **Fever---**lemon grass, apple cider vinegar sponge	**Gargle with lemon**-gargle bayberry tea **Cold or congestion lemon** grass* boil together 2-3 onions, 2-3 garlic bulbs (cut up)boil till tender in 1 qt. Water + pinch of cayenne- drink 4 ounces every 20 minutes **Chest cold:-**mullein, comfrey herbs -vapor with peppermint -mustard plaster over chest-1 cup of honey, ½ tsp. Peppermint oil, ½ tsp. Clove oil, ½ tsp. Cayenne, juice of 4 lemons,mix and take ½ tsp. As needed -mix 1 cup of olive oil, 6 tbs. Of cayenne pepper and ½ tbsp. Of peppermint oil. Apply over chest, cove with a hot pack daily **Cough –***heating compress to chest* -syrup- a.1cup honey, 1 garlic bulb, cut up 3-4 radishes , cut up1/2 tsp peppermint oil / eucalyptus ,juice of 3 lemons, pinch of ginger, pinch of cayenne (blend will tape 1/2 tsp as needed) **Head cold:-**vapor inhalation -chest congestion-hot foot bath-sweating wet sheet pack Hot foot bath with a little mustard -swear sheet pack **Sore throat**--see heating compress to throat -unset - see Russian steam bath Do chest fomentations - do hot foot bath-Epson salt bath (very hot) use 2 lbs. For 15 minutes- after go to bed and keep warm **Strep throat :** cayenne **Stuffy nose (**humidifier) heat lamp

COLIC

Note-Abnormal amounts of gas are passing upward or downward, and this is causing pain. *Colic babies* usually lasts 2-6 weeks- bottle fed babies have it more often-breast fed moms must be careful of diet (beans, cabbage, garlic, onion, chocolate, tuna, eggs, corn, wheat)- are contributors to colic	**Herb:-**catnip 1 tsp tea -peppermint 1tsp tea -1/4 of a bay leaf boiled for 15 minutes and drink - garlic oil - charcoal powder (1tbs in 4 oz. Water)-hops/ chamomile tea / catnip tea for babies -anise seed tea (bruise it by rubbing them together)

Cause: allergies to cow milk - various food in-takes of breastfeeding mother may cause colic- change to a vegan diet **Infant warm catnip tea** in a bottle. A catnip tea enema will also help. Crying spells occur at regular intervals; so, if a very warm bath is given an hour before an expected attack, it may be prevented. **Breast feeding mom**-<u>avoid-</u> onions, cabbage, garlic, wheat, yeast, broccoli, and Brussels sprouts, fried food, junk food, refined food, -breast fed infant points to the food given to the child. It may be the milk, wheat, soy, or sugar in the formula **Cleanse-** enemas daily for 3 days, babies 1-2 oz. Of warm water	Carob powder t thyme-bayberry - alfalfa , yellow sweet clover -2 parts fennel + 1 parts peppermint mix 1 tsp in 1 glass of water-ginger tea-with a little fructose for infants -caraway in milk or water for infants-bayberry tea, 1 tbs. Alfalfa mint, ½ tsp. Ginger tea mix in 1 pt. Water to make tea- drink 2 cups daily- produces relief from gas -chamomile in one glass water daily -1 bay leaf in a qt. Water -lemon water, vitamin-c-100-600 mg daily Drink lots of lemon water **To relax-**hops tea, catnip tea, chamomile tea **Enema-**glycerin suppository
COLITIS	
Symptoms: bloody diarrhea, bloody mucus, gas, pain, bloating, incomplete elimination of thebowels, weakness, weight loss, indiges-tion, headache, sometimes hard stoolulcerated colon **Causes:**-studies show that 70% of patients with this disease are lactose intolerance -cow's milk sensitivity -food allergies- take a pulse test <u>Avoid:</u>stress, worry, rush and-eggs, tomatoes, beef, coffee, condiments, spinach, citrus,- gluten (wheat, rye, barley, oats, buckwheat- very hot or cold foods or drinks (irritate the digestive tract)- more than 2-3 foods per meal-all animal products **Supplements-** 4 cap daily slippery elm -psyllium powder in glass of water or juice 3x daily -wheat grass- juice and sprouts -acidophilus- 6 caps daily-up to 1 tbs. Chia seed, ground, 2x daily in juice, capsules or water -1 tsp each skullcap, fireweed, hyssop, golden-seal, white oak bark in 1 qtr. Water- steep for ½ hr.- drink through the day –opt. Add sassafras, anise, fennel, wintergreens -Tea-flaxseed tea- 1tsp. In 1 cup boil water steep till gelatinous- drink at night	**Drinking charcoal slurry** **Bleeding-** yellow dock or burdock root tea – 1 tbsp. To 1 qt. Of water- enema-(4 times weekly) enemas (104-108 f.) Relieves pain **Raw cabbage** Drink fresh, carrot, celery and parsley juices, to help heal the colitis. **Enema-**a hot retention enema given at about 109 to 110 degrees of goldenseal tea and pectin mixed Give enema (garlic or coffee- 10oz. 1x daily) - hot enemas -may add bayberry tea1 tbs. To 1 qt. Water (115-122 degrees far) **Diet-** -½ cup aloe Vera gel daily-take 8 oz. Of freshly prepared cabbage juice -before each meal -liquid diet for a short time -high fiber, vegetar-ian diet, bland-eat additional bran-add crushed psyllium seeds to diet - eat acidophilus twice daily-drink 1 tbs. Blackstrap molasses in a cup of hot water-5 hours should be allowed between meals -do not use sugar substitute-colitis are frequently relieve by distilled water-take 8 oz. Freshly pre-pared cabbage juice before each meals High-fiber foods are very important, also drink-ing lots of water.

-pectin by mouth. Put one tablespoon of crude pectin (canning variety) in a cup of water and stir it. Take three doses per day.

-Two goldenseal capsules three times a day.

-Two enteric coated peppermint oil capsules as needed for abdominal cramping.

-One half teaspoon of licorice powder to one cup of water per day (for its salt retaining or steroidal effect).

-slippery elm tea, one teaspoon in one cup of very warm water. Take one cup three times a day at usual mealtimes even if skipping the meal.

-Alfalfa, myrrh, and pau d'arco. Garlic and papaya are also useful. Aloe Vera- two ounces once or twice daily just before meals,

-peppermint (3 or more cups daily), fennel, licorice, catnip, goldenseal and alfalfa, garlic , psyllium, slippery elm, aloe Vera , chamomile tea

-goldenseal- 1 tsp. And ¼ tsp. Myrrh to a pint of boiling water-(take 1 tbs. 6-8x daily)

-do not eat raw greens, carrots, or peanuts. Eat cooked or steamed green leafy vegetables, cooked white potatoes, multigrain bread, and well-cooked oat bran, brown rice, millet, sweet potatoes, bananas, cooked carrots, squash, and avocados.

-brown rice or rice water

Pain :hot foot bath with hot compress to abdomen

Hydrotherapy

-inflammation- charcoal compress made with strong hops tea instead of water (all night)

-take a bath , adding 3 cups of apple cider vinegar to the bath and 2 tbs. Of acidophilus (for 30 minutes)- add 3 tbs. Ginger in bath nightly

-hot steam bath 3x daily-hot charcoal pack nightly

-fomentations to the abdomen once a day for 20 minutes with a hot foot bath.

COLON

Note-toxins- most diseases are caused by a toxic colon

Herbs: best herb is*aloe, burnet

Pain-fireweed-fleabane-use as an enema

Wheat grass- retaining enema daily for 5 hours

Colon cleanses formula: 1/3 lb. Each of-Agar agar—apple fiber—alfalfa—psyllium—slippery elm—charcoal—Senna + 3 tsp. Mandrake + pinch of cayenne + wormwood 1/4 lb, (take 1 tbsp. In ¼ cup juice 5x daily

Colon bowel aid -2 cups chopped or ground up fruit (such as raisins, prunes, apricots, peaches, apples, dates or figs) 1 oz. Powdered slippery elm bark +1 oz. Powdered flax seed+ 1 oz. Powdered licorice root -Mix together. Then add Just enough sorghum/ blackstrap molasses to moisten the dry ingredients. Mix it well + mold into small bars. Then roll these in equal parts of Slippery Elm bark and carob powder so it is no longer sticky.

CONGESTION

Hydrotherapy

-*Head*- hot foot bath with a little mustard*alternate hot and cold to head

-*congestion of internal organs*- hot tub bath may add 2 cups of mustard powder to water

-*chest* - (mustard plaster)

-*body part*- see fomentation chest- steam inhalation

-*cerebral*- see wet sheet pack (heating stage)

-*nasal*- heating compress to chest ,fomentation, hot foot bath

-*menstrual*: - hot foot bath

-*organ congestions*: - ice bag to area

Herb:coltsfoot - 1/3 part cayenne+ ¼ part ginger + peppermint oil+ 1 cup honey

Chickweed, mullein, plantain, sorrel, white oak bark, bayberry bark, comfrey, eucalyptus leaves, white pine needles, and oregano.

-lungs - fomentation for chest congestion	

CONJUNCTIVITIS =*PINK EYE*

Allergic conjunctivitis - vitamin-c 1000-3000mg daily, quercetin 1000mg daily, cold compresses **Charcoal poultice** **Compress with any of these herbs:**-bilberry, aloe Vera, chickweed, eyebright, fennel, red raspberry, or slippery elm-put chamomile tea bag in warm (not hot) water for 2-3 minutes -squeeze andplace over eye for 2-3 minutes do this 3-4 times daily Gauze saturated with witch hazel place over closed eyelid for 15 minutes-relieves irritation-onion poultice -white potatoes poultice **Supplement:** vitamin-c 2000-10,000 mg daily, quertin **Saline irrigation**	**Eye drops:**-charcoal slurry - eye drops-boil 1cups of water + 1/4 tsp salt +1 tsp charcoal powder (put 4-5 drops in eye-every 2 hours-1/2 tsp. Lemon + 4 oz. Distilled water drop in eye- cover with a slice of onion that has been warmed in oven-cucumber slices **Hydrotherapy:** saline eyewash. Use one level teaspoon salt per pint water. **Charcoal poultice.** Put charcoal in cloth bag, or spread on a paper towel. Cover with plastic to prevent drying. Tape in place. **Ice compress:** every 2-3 minutes x 1/2 hours discontinue after 30-60 minutes-hot (2 minutes) and cold(30 sec.) Compress every 4 hours

CONSTIPATION

<u>Do not use Senna with piles, collapse intestine/rectum</u> **<u>Do not use mineral oi</u>l**: it causes decrease in vitamin d, a, k ,and e, which leads to cancer **To train bowel:**- use ear irrigation bulb and fill with cold water and give self an enema hold water for 1 minutes (use it at the same time daily) **Constipation in children**- 1 oz. Raspberry leaves + ½ oz. Flaxseed **Irregular bowel movements:** flaxseed, plantain, Senna -take magnesium 400-800mg every night before bed, diatomaceous earth 1 tbs. Daily	**Impaction:-** liquid acidophilus- 1/2 bottle oil retention enema overnight **Eat prunes or figs.** Flaxseed meal (best freshly ground) is helpful. **Remove accumulated fecal** matter—large hot enema or hot colonic; neutral enema; oil retention (oil enema to be retained throughout the night). Repeat till bowel is thoroughly emptied, and then inject a pint of water at 75^0-70^0 f., to tone the bowel. **Pain:** -fennel ginger -drink a glass of water every 10 minutes until the bowels move

CONVULSION INFANTILE

Avoid cow's milk if curds are present in the stools. Daily cold bath, wet hand rub, or cold towel rubs. **Alternate hot and cold** pail pours, if necessary. Apply hot abdominal pack, changing every 4 hours.	**For immediate relief**, hot blanket pack; warm bath, at 95^0-98^0 f., for 1-2 minutes. If not quickly relieved, remove from bath and employ cold pail pour to head and spine. **Give a large** hot enema

COUGH

Quick set of *three revulsive* to chest (two minutes hot, twenty seconds cold), hot foot bath	**Lemon juice**+ honey +a pinch of cayenne - use 1 tsp. As needed

Heating compresses to chest overnight. Place a thin washcloth or a t-shirt squeezed from ice water on the chest. Cover entirely with one inch to spare on all sides with one of the following: a thick piece of wool or synthetic pinned in place, or plastic piece cut from a bread bag. Dress warmly in a sweater. When removing, sponge chest with cold water or alcohol.-fomentation to spine

Sipping hot water -gargling hot water- several times each day

Copious water drinking is best

Steam inhalation- with few drops of eucalyptus oil or peppermint oilbreath for 10- 15 minutes- 3-4x daily

Cold compress to throat

Antispasmodic tincture

-lobelia tincture 1 0z -skullcap tincture 1 oz. -skunk cabbage tincture (if available)-1 oz. -myrrh tincture 1 oz. -black cohosh tincture 1 oz. - cayenne pepper 1 tsp

-(mix give 8-15 drops in 1/2 glass water- if can't drink place under tongue)

Herbs-use same herbs + 1 qtr. Boiling water- let stand x 1 hour- strain -add 1 pt. Honey-put under low heat let it evaporate to 3 cups-use 1 tsp for cough, asthma, convulsions, insomnia

Pinch of ginger- pinch of cayenne pepper (blend well and take 1-2 tsp as

Needed)

Boil 1 qt. Water + 1/2tsp. Cayenne wrap hot mixture around neck in towel –change hot fomentation every 3-4 minutes-hot foot bath

Tea-1 oz. Thyme+ ½ oz. Mouse ear +1oz. Glycerin+ dash cinnamon- in 1 qt. H20 pour hot h20 cover let cool- take 1 tsp for coughing prn(brings up phlegm)

Cough syrup: mix two tablespoons honey, two tablespoons water, and a drop of eucalyptus—as much as will stay on a toothpick.

-1cup honey, ½ tsp cayenne, ½ tsp peppermint oil, 1/3 cup fructose

-chop 1 onion put in glass jar + ½ cup lemon juice put next to window expose to sun light

-1 cup honey, 1/2cup fructose, juice of 3 lemons, 1 cup garlic, ½ tsp cayenne, 1/3 tsp. Peppermint oil, 1/3 tsp. Clove oil, blend and refrigerate

Child cant cough up phlegm- burn cayenne in skillet

Make a cough syrup for children (pour 1 qtr. Of water over the above herbs(no vinegar or alcohol)- let stand x1 hour then strain- add 1 pint of honey-place over low heat let it evaporate to 2 cupful's seal in small jars-2 dry figs to a glass of soy milk and bring to a boil- allow to stand for an hour, warm up and drink all at once 2x daily

COUGH whooping

contagious bacterial isolate from other children

Attacks children between 6 months to 5 years

Complications: -convulsions -bleeding nose, brain, around eye;

Broncho-pneumonia

Severe cough: -drink warm water- one cup after another

- then stick your finger down his throat and have him vomit-after vomit -rinse mouth to prevent- Damage of teeth from hydrochloric acid

Copious drinking of hot water

Place him on a full fruit juice fast **Herb-***Wild cherry bark tea is excellent*-slippery elm tea with lemon= excellent

Roast onions or fry them and apply to chest and back

Fomentation to spine; sipping hot water

It is good to soak the feet in hot water, with a little mustard and salt added to it

-Put oil on bottom of child's feet (poultice of garlic) grease the bottom of his feet with grease (petroleum) make 1/4 inch thick put on soft cloth put on bottom of each feet and put socks on do morning and evening	*For painful cough:* Fomentation to chest every 2 hours **Relieve cough**—chest and neck heating pack, changing every 4 hours

CROUP

Description- harsh barking cough with high pitch respiratory sound it is often associated with the 1st or 4th night of measles often caused by overeating*check for allergies* **Croup can be caused by bacteria or viruses.** —The larynx (vocal cords) or trachea (wind-pipe) narrows frequently affects children from 3 months to 3 years (9 to 18 months is the peak) **Maintain a good water intake** **Hot onion pack** to chest and back 3x daily- place sliced onion between clothes and cover with heating pad **Carrot juice**-do not give milk –use quinoa (blend and make as a milk after cooking) **Verywarm ginger herb** bath- then wrap him in towel put him to bed and let him perspire **Cold washcloth or ice pack** around the neck, with a dry towel on top, keep neck cold till swelling is gone - increase water intake (lukewarm) **Carob tea** -rice water enema 1x daily **Peppermint oil -1 1/3 tsp. In 1 cup**	*To relieve spasm:* hit the chest with end of a cold wet towel or dash of cold water over chest and back If spasm is severe, -relieve the congestion by hot blanket pack or hot full bath. Repeat every 3-6 hours. Hot half bath with cold pail pour to head, back, and chest. Follow bath with ice-cold heating compress to neck, change every 2-4 hours. Fomentation to cervical, upper, and middle spine for 15 minutes each time the ice compress is changed. **Honey and lemon,** ½ tsp. Cayenne- mix and take ½tsp. As needed **Lemon and honey** 1 spoonful at a time every 15 minutes Peppermint and honey + few drops of lobelia in catnip tea or chamomile tea -give catnip tea enema **Teas:** -Echinacea, fenugreek, goldenseal, thyme, ginger **Warm vaporizer** at night-cold water wrung out t- shirt + hot sweater over wet t- shit for at least 8hours -neck + upper chest fomentation-fomentation to throat for 15 min., every 2 hours

CUSHING'S (adrenal over-activity)

Symptoms:-rounded moon face-heavy abdomen and buttocks, thin extremities Eyelids may appear swollen and round-red spots may appear in the face- Poor wound healing and skin thinness (leading to stretch marks and easily bruising)-peptic ulcers hypertension, diabetes, mental instability may also occur scalp balding, brittle bones, body hair grows faster. Women may grow mustache and beards-healing more difficult, illness is more frequent -causes kidney stone formation, dizziness	*Hydrotherapy*--hot Epson salt bath nightly (3 tbs. Per bath) -drink 2-3 qt. Water daily *Take*--**no enema cleanser** daily- **enema** 2x daily **Alfalfa**-5tabs 5xdaily -chlorophyll- 4 oz. 2x daily-green drink- 1 pt. Or more **Multi vitamins daily** -calcium 800-1000 mg daily -vitamin-e 600-1000mg daily B-complex 600mg daily -vitamin-c 500- 2000mg daily -kelp- 6 caps 2x daily -cleanse Licorice 5 caps 3x daily-wild yam -2 caps 2x daily(-200mg daily

Cause:- of corticosteroid hormones overdose (especially from those used to treatrheumatism and arthritis)-the outer rind of the adrenal gland which is located on top of each kidney produces cortisone malfunctions	
CYANOSIS	
Description- skin s bluish due to lack of oxygen	**Hydrotherapy:** -hot blanket pack for 15 minutes- followed by cold-mitten friction- avoid chill
CYSTS POLYPS	
Research high vitamin C diet.	Garlic, burdock, goldenseal, red clover,
CYSTIC FIBROSIS	
Symptoms:-1st seen in very small children, large amount of thick mucus develops inlungs, chronic coughing, wheezing and lung infection, blocking lung passages, , digestive problems, inadequate absorption of fats, after meal, stomach pain, thinness, body sweat will have a very large amount of sodium, potassium, and chloride, salts (any / all of these symptoms may occur) **Causes:**- it is an inherited disease which causes-inadequate absorption of selenium, zinc,essential fatty acids, and other minerals including trace minerals, leading toceliac disease (inability to tolerate wheat and other foods)	**Supplements:**-safflower- able to remove hard phlegm from the system-germanium - in garlic and onions, selenium, vitamin-E **Herbs:** Echinacea, licorice root, ginger, yarrow, peppermint, cayenne, garlic, mullein Include germanium (found in garlic and onions), selenium, and vitamin E.

DEBILITY

Increase endurance: Tonic frictions, which include Wet Hand Rub, Cold Mitten Friction, Cold Towel Rub, Wet Sheet Rub, Dripping Sheet Rub, Ice Rub, and Salt Glow. *In cases of severe exhaustion*, bed rest , proper diet, plus carefully graduated tonic cold applications, Percussion Douche to spine

Take one gallon of good wholesome grape juice. Add a cup of raisins which are high iron. Add a cup of *apricots*, which is one of the highest sources of iron and is the most easily assimilated form. Then add one cup of *figs*. Put at least a half cup *black strap molasses* + 5 Tbsp. Of *Black Cherry* concentrate also. Sit overnight on the counter. The next morning put it in the refrigerator. Drink about 4 ounces 3 or 4 times a day, depending on how low your hemoglobin is. This will bring it up within thirty days.

Tonic tea-1 oz. Wild cherry bark, 2t flax seed, 1 lemon juice+ 1 qt. H20 steep- 1 glassful daily.

Formula tonic tea-Comfrey 1 tbs. + red clover 3 tbsp. + alfalfa mint 2 tbs.+ horsetail 1 tbsp.,

Mix all together, use 2 tbs. In 1 pt., of water-make tea and take 3 cups daily

Mix together 1 oz. Parsley root, 1 oz. Alfalfa; 1/2 oz. Of each of the following: dandelion root, yellow dock root, comfrey root, burdock root, nettles leaves, and dulse. Place in an uncovered pot with a quart of water and simmer for 20 minutes, Let cool, then strain. Place the liquid back in the pot and simmer uncovered for one hour or till it is reduced to one cup. Stir in one cup of unsulphured blackstrap molasses and refrigerate. Take one tablespoonful 3 times daily.

DEPRESSION

Causes:-loss of loved one/ job, environmental problems -food allergies, post-menstrualsyndrome -severe illness/ stroke -twice more common in female than male-lack of niacin causes deep depression -hypoglycemia,-b12 deficiency causes depression -high sugar diet produces depression

200 medicinal drugs are reported to cause depression -birth control pills-steroids, corticosteroids -diet pills -low protein diet, house dust, perfume, formaldehyde, and cosmetics as allergenic factors to be avoided. Low blood sugar induces depression

Cocktail: ounces of liquid extracted from juicer-beet tops 2oz. ,parsley 2 oz., spinach 2 oz., carrots 6 oz., 1/2 tomatoes(mix and drink daily)

Herbal and vitamin treatments: mix together-sage, catnip and alfalfa and make into a tea, take 1 cup every am and pm-*pasque flower* mix with mint, linden blossoms, skullcap anise and fennel (take 3 cupsdaily for 1 months)

Take gava

Hydrotherapy-avoid very hot or prolonged cold baths; /cold to head when face is

Supplement- *lecithin* 1 tbsp. 3x daily- black strap molasses 1 tbsp. 3x daily- vitamin-b6 100mg 3x daily-vitamin-b12 1000mcg daily- magnesium 800mg daily- potassium 99mg 5x daily-olive oil 1 tbs. 2x daily, noni

Balanced amino acids, especially tyrosine and taurinepale.

DIABETIC

Parasites are one of the causes of diabetes(especially in children) and hypothyroidism-stress, oral contraceptives, drugs, adrenal corticosteroids, phenytoin-thiazide, high sugar and white flour diet

Herbal-take-a=acute; sa=subacute; c=chronic; d=degenerative

Sugar---use stevia-

Formula: gymnemasylvestre, jambul seed, huckleberry leaves, horsetail, couch grass, uvaursi, princess pine

Garlic per day proven to lower blood sugar

Sa(hypoglycemia) juniper, kelp, licorice root. Safflower

C-(diabetes) blueberry leaves, juniper berry, goldenseal

-*banana leaf extract* 45mg 3 divided doses daily

Cedar berries helps the pancreas- devil's club, dandelion burdock

-*cinnamon extract* as directed -huckleberry-helps promote insulin production

Diet-lots of raw garlic, lots of raw onion, eat buckwheat, rice, corn which have no gluten, 75% raw, 10 % cooked, 10% protein, 3 % nuts fat free diet proven to lower blood sugar, eating hastily increases blood, sugar levels, eliminate alcohol and caffeine, nitrites in meat increases blood sugar, alkaline diet

-avoid gluten foods (wheat, rye, oats, barley)

-*string beans* tea 1cup 3x daily 1cup= 1unit of insulin

-*onions* has been used for centuries to treat diabetes

-*squeeze juice out of a wholegrapefruit* then simmer in 3 ½ glass of water for 15 minutes- take 1 glass ½ hour before each mea

-*juice cilantro and cucumber* 3x daily heals pancreas

Low blood sugar-dandelion coffee -huckleberry tea -blueberry tea -chick pea roasted coffee-lecithin 2 tbsp. Daily

Goldenseal if taking add = amount of licorice root to it-*otherwise diabetics with high sugar should not take licorice*

Gurmar- used to treat diabetes -dandelion- contains insulin like compounds-fenugreek

Herbs-blueberry/ huckleberry leaf tea 1cup 3x daily-goldenseal 4cap 3x daily for 1 week -black walnut 1tsp 2x daily-juniper berries chewed up to 6-8 berries 2x daily or goldenseal up to 20 capsules daily-lecithin 1 tsp 2x daily

-*string beans* tea 1cup 3x daily 1cup= 1unit of insulin

-vanadyl sulfate 100-150mg daily

-chromium 200-300mg daily -veradium 100mcg daily

-*fenugreek*-six compounds which help regulate blood sugar levels

Herbs-wild squash powder -soybean coffee once daily -agar 1 tbsp. In juice daily-licorice root 7cap 2x daily -lecithin 1 tsp. 2x daily

Herbs-yarrow, mugwort, shepherd purse, mariola, thyme, bilberry white oak, poplar, St. John's wort, witch hazel, - carob powder 1 tsp 2x daily -raw garlic, -barley green -take esiac tea -huckleberry leaf= cures mild diabetes=natural insulin -bitter melon- good

Neurolaenalobata-ten gm.

Regular exercise is key

DIARRHEA

Diarrhea in infants -can be checked by the use of thin *rice or barley water*. For an older child, use *oatmeal gruel*. This should be given until the looseness is checked.

Chronic diarrhea, electrolyte and trace mineral deficiencies are likely. Rice water, lime water, *potato broth,* and fruit will help restore lost electrolytes.

Alternating constipation and diarrhea—large warm (98⁰ f.) Enema or colonic, once or twice a week; follow with a small cold enema and hot abdominal pack

Mucous stools—large hot enema at 95⁰ f., followed by small cold enema; cold compress to abdomen, changed every hour; revulsive sitz bath or revulsive compress to abdomen; revulsive fan douche to abdomen.

Pain in abdomen with tenderness—fomentation to abdomen every 2-3 hours; hot enema at 100⁰ f., after each bowel movement; heating compress over abdomen after each hot application, to be changed once an hour until the

Dysentery (acute), colitis —dietary needs—free water drinking, a simple dietary with no animal broths or meat preparations. Fresh ripe fruit, brown rice, and fruit juices, with well-cooked cereals.

Dysentery (chronic), colitis (chronic) rest in bed; careful diet; graduated cold baths, twice daily; cold rubbing sitz bath; hot revulsive sitz bath 6-10 minutes daily, immediately preceded by a hot enema.

Pain-if much pain is present, revulsive sitz bath once or twice a day. Moist abdominal bandage.

Cleanse colon by large hot enema daily

Frequent stools—abdominal compress as above; prolonged cool sitz bath at 75⁰ f., 15 minutes, followed by short hot pail pour to spine and wet sheet rub,

Next hot application is made.

Helpful herbs include *white oak bark* blackberry, plantain, barley, clove root, whortleberry, black currant, burdock, and Echinacea. Dried blueberries.

Charcoal/ clay is also useful in stopping diarrhea

Diet-aseptic dietary, especially fruit juices, purees, well-cooked cereals.

-Straight *lemon or lime juice*, taken on an empty stomach

-Cook down *apple peels* and drink it

DIPHTHERIA

Each day, clean all clothing and bed linens by boiling them.

Do not give aspirin to a child or youth with a fever; it may result in death! **Symptoms:**-begins with sore throat and fever-difficulty swallowing, hoarseness-frequently a dirty, white ,grayish membrane forms in the throat +/ nose(may beyellowish or green) -children-unevenly, swollen, red tonsils-swollen neckglands-throat-grey film and nose-vomit, hoarse, tonsillitis call an M.D this is a life-threatening disease -danger- membrane obstruct breathing, the germ causes

Heart muscle, nerves and kidney damage -transmitted by animals, clothes, raw

Milk, contact individuals can carry the germs for years and transmit it

Membrane forms in the throat or nose, or both.

Symptom-There are slight chills, possible vomiting and diarrhea, always fetid breath, difficulty in swallowing, and hoarseness. Children first complain of feeling tired and sleepy. The tonsils appear dark red, inflamed and unevenly swollen. White, parchment-like patches appear on them. The glands in the neck often swell.

Suffocation-threatened suffocation—put him in a neutral full bath at 102⁰-105⁰ f. And pours cold water over the chest and spine. Cold mitten friction.

Tissue sloughing (heating compress 60f.) Changing every hour-**antispasmodic tincture:**-lobelia 1 oz.-skullcap 1 oz. -skunk cabbage 1 oz. -myrrh 1 oz.-black cohosh 1 oz.-1/2 oz. Cayenne powder -juice of 5 lemons -garlic bulb juiced- drink 3 oz. 3x daily

Emetic- An emetic is usually needed, to empty the stomach of putrefying matter; Lobelia in water can be given, but combined with bayberry bark is better. (may add small amount of cayenne and ginger) *The vomiting must be repeated* until the stomach and throat are entirely clean. *As the disease progresses,* lobelia and bayberry bark tea may be given at any time, to clean out the mucous membranes of the mouth and throat. Bayberry cleans the membrane and eliminates the odor. A very small amount of ginger or cayenne can be added

Problems can develop while the child is sleeping—serious ones. Always give him the emetic before he goes to sleep each time. Otherwise possible suffocate in his sleep.

Give the child all the water he can drink, and keep him in bed or may overstrain the heart. In a well-ventilated room. Avoid chilling him. Too early exercise

If properly cared for, the disease will end within 7-10 days.

Diet: -lots of fluid -fast of fresh carrot juice or fresh citrus juices. -bananas, raisins, figs, oranges-no meat

If the child insists on eating something, *give him bananas, raisins, figs, and oranges* and no other food. It is best to give him only liquids (water and fresh juices) until he is cleaned out, the throat is clean, and the phlegm and false membrane are totally gone. When the disease appears to be ended, give no meat at all.

As he begins to recuperate, he can be given baked apples, potato peeling broth, fresh fruits, cooked vegetables, and soy milk.

Hydrotherapy- Give him warm baths.

Paralysis—fomentation to spine with short hot blanket or cold mitten friction pack, followed by cold mitten friction; hot and cold friction over the affected part; gymnastics; massage; and appropriate exercise.

Give him an enema *every morning and evening.* This helps clean out toxins from the diphtheria germs. An herb tea can be added to detoxify colon: bayberry, white oak bark, or red raspberry. There should be at least 3-4 movements a day.

Heart failure-symptoms of heart failure: -1/2 tsp. Of cayenne in hot water- drink all immediately

Herbal:- cayenne, ginger or bayberry and gingko-gargle lemon juice every 1/2 hour andswallow-give lobelia (1ts. In hot water) with bayberry bark emetic add a little ginger/cayenne-gargle - goldenseal + myrrh with pinch cayenne

Mucus- Bayberry is excellent in all **throat or stomach mucous** conditions. -A garglecan be made of goldenseal and myrrh, with a pinch of cayenne. Use this every half hour. It will clean the mucous and germs out of the throat.

DIVERTICULITIS

Check stools: -if black= bleeding

Symptom:-chills, fever, pain localized in the left, lower quadrant-if you are over 40 and have periodic abdominal cramps, gas, diarrhea alternating -with constipation, you may have diverticulitis

Cause:- constipation, and too much protein, refined carbohydrates, animal fats study shows*high fat*diet to be a cause-

During an attack- give yourself a

-*cleansing enema* (2 quarts of water and the juice of a fresh lemon).

-*Take 4 charcoal* tablets with a large glass of water. If pain or spasm in the colon, apply a heating pad over the abdomen.

-*eat a low-fiber diet* for a short time. Then return to the high-fiber regime. **S-***blend* food, carrots, cabbage, green juices

Clay decreases inflammation of the diverticulum(sac-like areas which balloon from the colon)

Helpful herbs include slippery elm, peppermint, chamomile, and aloe Vera-1-2 tbsp. Crushed flaxseed 2-3x daily with lots of water-slippery elm- prunes-chamomile tea-paud'arco- 2 cups daily - aloe Vera, goldenseal, cayenne, yarrow,papaya, red clover-psyllium seed- 1tsp. With 8 oz. Water or juice taken at meals-garlic

Formula: wild yam- 2 parts, valerian- 1 part, black haw - 1 part peppermint -1 part

Supplement: b-complex, acidophilus, beta carotene, (25,000 iu.) Daily, vitamin-e (600iu)daily-vitamin-c with bioflavonoids (200mg) in divided doses

Carrot, beet, celery, and green juices Are excellent. Of the fruit juices, papaya, apple, pineapple, and lemon are outstanding for your purposes. **Wheat grass juice retention** enemas-retain for 20 minutes	**Diet-**Chew nuts, seeds, and popcorn well, so they will be less likely to enter the diverticula. Eat smaller meals. Low high-fat diets, for 90 week Avoid caffeine +sugar products. They all tend to irritate the colon.

DIZZINESS(VERTIGO)

Check for: -b6 and niacin and magnesium deficiency-brain tumors, high or low blood pressure, viral infection -middle ear infection, uses of certain drugs, excess wax -blockage of ear canal/ Eustachian tube -vertigo = warning sign of coming heart attack/ stroke -too much sodium disrupts the operation of the inner ear **If the cause** is low-blood pressure, lower your head while the blood gets up there. **Supplement**-niacin, B_6, and the entire B complex—including B_1, B_2, and pantothenic acid. Vitamin C. **Do not take over** 2,000 mg of total sodium per day. Too much sodium disrupts the operation of the inner ear. Take powdered peppercorns, onion.	**Catnip tea will help** **Swedish bitters**- moisture cloth and apply to head-need cleanse **Herbs:** gingko*- , lemon balm, ginger- seasick, celery seed, catnip tea, cayenne – 3 cap daily **Supplements**: b- complex- especially B6, B1, pantothenic acid, vitamin E , lecithin, niacin-100mg 2x daily, acidophilus 10 capsules daily, magnesium 1000mg daily, calcium 1000mg daily, garlic 10 tablets daily (or eat raw garlic), ginkgo 3 caps 3x Daily , vitamin C (5000mg daily), **Hydrotherapy:-**fomentations to the stomach followed by hot abdominal packs -bathe face or top of head with very hot water or hot compress for 2 minutes- followed by cool compress for 15 minutes -heat to back of neck in anemia of the brain

DUMPING SYNDROME

Take English bitters, along with folic acid, pectin, and eat as carefully as you can. Take full vitamin/mineral supplementation.	Lie down for half an hour after each meal

DYSLEXIA

-food allergy is a key problem -beware of sugar, wheat and certain, other grains, milk ("pot" to "top") or reverse ("b" for "d")	**-take hydrochloric** acid for a while (betaine HCL) and digestive enzymes Carry out pulse tests (see allergy section) (which see), to determine possible causes

EAR

Do not place liquid or oil in the ear if you think the drum has burst. *If this pus starts leaking to the outside,* then the eardrum has ruptured.

Herbal-a=acute; sa=subacute; c=chronic; d=degenerative ear

A-earache) mullein, lobelia, garlic, Echinacea

Sa- (earwax) garlic oil

C-(hard of hearing) plantain, rue, cloves

D-(deafness) blue violet, cayenne (stimulates circulation)

Earache hydrotherapy-hot and cold to ear, heat to face, hot water gargle for ten minutes, head and neck kept warm when out-of-doors, ice pack to throat, and fasting one or two meals. Use fruits and juices at regular mealtimes when not fasting.

-*alleviate pain in the ear,* use a little olive oil or garlic oil in the ear, and then add a drop or two of lobelia tincture. Or

-*make a paste,* using *onion powder or clay packs.* Then apply this to the outside of the ear.

-*Bake a large onion until it becomes soft,* and tie it over the ear; this will often give great relief for pain is severe.

Ear oil of garlic-Dosages: With an eye dropper put into each ear at night four to six drops of oil of garlic and four to six drops of the herb tincture listed below plugging ears overnight with cotton, do this six days a week, four to six months, or as needed. On the seventh day, flush ears with a small ear syringe using warm apple cider vinegar and distilled water half and half.

-*ear oil:* 1 garlic clove in 1/3 cup olive oil in glass jar and shake daily x 2 weeks – keep refrigerated

Earwax:- Hearing loss with no ear pain =possible wax build up

H2o2- or mineral oil or glycerin in the ear -flush ear body-temperature- gentlysqueeze in ear with head tilted and let - water flow out

1 part warm water+ 1 part vinegar in ear -few drops of h2o2 in ear -garlic oil 1-2 days

-vitamin-C 500mg 3x daily after 6 months. Ear will not produce wax-*ear candle*

Hearing loss:-mullein oil

Infection-Place drops of hydrogen peroxide in the ear, to help clean it out. Then rinse out with water. Do not leave the peroxide there.

Garlic -cut a clove of garlic leave skin- put in effected ear

Insect in ear:- piece of ripe apple or pear next to ear

Ringing in the ears (tinnitus), loss of balance, and severe dizziness

-Vitamin c. Calcium, vitamins a, b complex (including b_6, niacin, and pantothenic acid), manganese/ magnesium deficiency causes deafness need a low-salt diet. Eliminate-(milk, eggs, corn, wheat, and yeast)

-Mix 1 tsp. Salt and 1 tsp. Glycerin in 1 pint warm water. Several times a day, using a nasal sprayer, spray each nostril until it begins draining into the back of the throat; also spray the throat

-Variations in glucose levels can prompt Meniere's. Use one bowl for hot water and one for cold, once or twice a day, and take a hot and cold head bath. Immerse the head in the hot, for 30-60 seconds, and then plunge it into ice cold. (if elderly, weakened, or with a heart condition, begin with less extreme temperatures.)

-herbs which may help include cayenne, gotu kola, garlic, butcher's broom, ginkgo balboa, and ginger. At the time of an attack, lying quietly on the affected side, with eyes turned in the direction of the affected ear may help reduce the immediate crisis.

-put cotton ball soaked in *Swedish bitters* in the ear

Swimmers ear: hydrogen peroxide-1oz.rubbing alcohol+ 1oz. Vinegar

Poultice:- charcoal poultice -clay poultice to back of ear 3x daily -*hot roasted onion toear -rub feet with olive oil then spread garlic over feet-place cotton ball soaked with Swedish bitters in ear

ECZEMA- rash	
-Usually allergy–check calcium deficiency Avoid dairy products, white flour, fried foods, other processed fats, and sugar,*Wheat gluten*, eggs, peanuts, milk, wheat, fish, chicken, pork, or beef. Eggs, peanuts, and milk account for 75 percent of the skin rashes in children	**Mix goldenseal root** powder with vitamin E oil and put some on the affected area. This will reduce the itching **Zinc-** clears eczema

EDEMA *dropsy/ swelling*	
Description- water accumulation under skin **Check-for-** kidneys, congestive heart failure varicose veins, phlebitis, protein, thiamine deficiency sodium retention , cancer, food allergy, hypothyroidism, anemia, adrenal, constipation, lack of exercise=deficiency of vitamin b1,3,6- *poor circulation because of liver and heart problemsis common* **Causes:** get a diagnosis before you can treat-lack of exercise –deficiency of vitamin-b complex, b1,b3, b6 and potassium-poor kidney function –congestive heart failure, varicose veins, protein andthiamine deficiency –liver disease –sodium retention –cancer-pregnancy, standing too long, oral contraceptives, allergy, injury **Remove lemon skin-** cut fruit into small pieces and cover with honey use one lemon juice per day gradually increase to 8 lemons	**Herbs:** corn silk, dandelion, Scotch broom, alfalfa, Canadian fleabane, garlic, English hawthorn, juniper berries, lily of the valley, parsley, nettle, marshmallow, pau d'arco, and prickly, hyssop tea, corn silk, dandelion, scotch broom, alfalfa, Canadian fleabane, garlic,English hawthorn, juniper berries, lily of the valley, parsley, nettle, marshmallow, pau d'arco, prickly ash **Increase vitamin-B6** intake to decrease fluid retention *Hydrotherapy-* alternate bath (add 2 cups salt to water), wet sheet pack (heating stage) *-abdomen-* alternate compress- h To tub bath 2x daily *-Chest* -alternate compress *-Legs:* contrast bath- painful- continuous hot shower **Swedish bitters-** 1 tbs. Am and pm

EMPHYSEMA	
Symptom: continual breathlessness, most any exertion brings cough, distended neck, veins, rapid short breathing **Eliminate pollutant --**smoking, etc. **Diet-**avoid gas forming foods which causes abdominal distention and interfere withbreathing (example-legumes , cabbage)-eat less a little more often-low salt diet -avoid hard to chew food -drink Enough water (helps clear mucus) -maintain ideal body weight **Eliminate congestion:-**hang from the waist over the edge of the bed with a bowl at the head for easyexpectoration-apply a hot, moist compress	**Hot and cold chest pack-** alternate hot and cold showers, cayenne **Hydrotherapy-** place a plastic sheet on top sheet and beneath the top sheet cover-dip a sheet in very cold water- wrap around the standing naked patient (except head)-wrap a dry blanket around him -put in bed and cover with plastic and top cover The effect is immediate freezing cold, which the body gradually warms. The person can remain like this all night. -<u>do not use</u> on frail thin people* **Herbs:** mullein, licorice, peppermint, elecampane **Flax seed oil-** decreases lung inflammation **Exercise:** -regular program a must

to the back repeatedly for 5-10 minutes-then have a friend pound vigorously on the back with palms open-as mucus loosen spit it out (repeat 1-3 times)	**Other helps:** -avoid constipation -fresh air -elevate head of bed-<u>avoid</u> perfume, animals, humid climate, gas stoves, carpeting, curtain draperies

ENDOCRINE-Herb-ho-shou-wu

ENDOMETRIOSIS

Symptoms:-abdominal pain, back pain, pelvic pain, bladder problems, bleeding problems, bleedingbetween periods, very painful menstrual cramps -in 30 % cases there is no symptoms **Causes-** tampons, internal contraceptives, sex during menstruation-there is hereditary factor -internal fetal monitors *Hydrotherapy*-hot fomentation to lower abdomen-ice bag or heating pad to lower abdomen orlower back -hot and cold sitz bath-for 20-30 min with hot foot bath at the same time-conclude with cold mitten rub -hot footbath for 30 minutes. Conclude all treatment with a cold mitten friction. *Take*-**vitamin/ mineral supplement**s -B- vitamin supplement-vitami-C (1,000-2,000mg) daily ' -vitamin-E(400-800 iu. Daily) -calcium (2,000 mg daily)-magnesium (2,000 mg daily) -potassium (5,500mg daily)	*Diet-* **eliminate:** -hormones -antibiotics -sugars, white flour products (contribute to Endometriosis) -meat, eggs, dairy products -drink carrot juice daily -flaxseed oil 2 tsp. Daily **Herbs:** black cohosh, Echinacea, goldenseal, cayenne, black cohosh, burdock, alfalfa tea, red raspberry tea Each month before the anticipated beginning of the menstrual **symptoms lessens** during pregnancy and lactation -Tampons reduce the internal flow and can increase the likelihood of developing or increasing the implants. They also increase pain and cramping. Women with endometriosis frequently have a difficult time getting pregnant turn and continues until menopause

EPILEPSY-*Brain electrical disturbance*

When attack is threatened:-give antispasmodic herbal formula -colonic twice daily-neutral pack -ice to head -rest in bed -place person in cold water (may avert the seizure) **After attack:**-rest, cold to head -cold mitten friction of cold towel rub-revulsive douche- spray to legs, and percussion douche to spine **Put compress** of Swedish bitters on back of head + drink 4 cups of stinging nettle, add 2 tbs. To tea of Swedish bitters daily- take for *months till healed* **Herbs-**hoary puccoon- Indians used the herb on persons thought to be near convulsion -valerian root, rosemary, mistle toe, lobelia	**Antispasmodic tincture**-rub on infants neck, chest, and between shoulders -place 2-3 drops in mouth and washdown with tsp. Of warm water in bed (repeat every 1-2 hours if necessary) **Keep bowels moving** (take lemon enema at night if no bowel movement For the day) (juice of 2 lemons in 2 qt. Water) **Children with convulsions-** give catnip enema, hawthorn, lily of the valley, lobelia tincture*blue vervain, gotu kola*passion flower, avoid sage **Epilepsy in babies-** shinleaf*** **Supplement:**-vitamin-b-1,a, vitamins, manganese -vitamin-D (1000mg) -folic acid (5mg) -zinc (30 mg)-aurine (an amino acid) -manganese (25mg)-magnesium-(1000mg)

Formula: mix 2 oz. Skullcap: 1 oz. Valerian root: and 1/4 oz. Each cayenne and lobelia- sift theherbs (at an attack give 1 tsp in a cup of hot water- every hour if necessary)	-avoid folic acid in excess of 400mcg per day(can trigger seizures)

EXTREMITIES (limbs)

See Reynaud's **Burning feet-**could be nerve inflammation A lack of niacin (a B vitamin) is a specific deficiency factor.- may affect other parts of body-add *niacin and niacinamide* to your diet Check allergies chemicals used in leather -b-complex, b1, b2, b6, b12 vitamins -drink brewer's yeast stirred up in water ;Add niacin -*cold compress* to area and change it every 20-30 minutes -cool or cold foot bath **Cramps leg**: need mg and potassium **Odor foot-** Soak your feet (15 minutes, twice a week) in ½ cup vinegar added to 1 quart of water. Soak them in alternate hot and cold water pans or pails. Caution if diabetic or have impaired circulation, Sprinkle some dry, crumbled sage leaves into your shoes, to control odor. *Sweating feet*: Revulsive Douche to the feet, with extremes in temperature as great as possible. Give an Alternate hot and cold Foot Bath. During the night, apply a Heating Compress to the feet; and give a Cold Mitten Friction to the feet in the morning, on arising **Swelling feet:**-hot salt water *soaks = parts, white oak bark,* wormwood, shave grass-steep 1tbs in1/2 cup of water--take in tsp doses -elevate feet -roll your feet over tennis ball or a rolling pin internally	**Frostbite:** can result in peeling and blistering, 24-72 hours later and perhaps cold sensitivity to area *Regular care:*-*roll self* in a ball to conserve energy-do <u>not</u> take off shoes-do <u>not</u>*rub ice* to area-instead rub area with cold water or snow -do <u>not</u> use *heat lamp*, hot water bottles, hair dryer-it causes burns -*cover warmly*-get in hot tub 100-110 degrees no more than 110-give warm liquids -paint on do <u>not</u>rub in olive oil, if infected paint on honey -sponge area with water from boil *potatoes* -sponge area with warm water -gently rub skin with *raw onions*, potatoes slices, or raw *radish* that has been liquefied *Severe cases:* with blisters-wrap area with gauze so blisters do not break-elevate legs -do not rub blisters-immerse legs in warm water and massage gently for 5-10 minutes Crafter being treated for frostbite:-daily 4 times a day apply *aloe Vera gel to* area (use from cut leaves if available)-or apply the inner sides of *cucumber peeling* -diet- high protein, with plenty of grains **Cold extremities:**-check for sluggish thyroid-B-complex vitamins, niacin, B2-put feet in cold water for 1 minute then jump rope, run or walk for 1-2 minutes - do that 3-4x

EYE

<u>Urgent-</u>*retina detached* - sudden appearance of *spots, strings eye,* -*floating, flashes* of light, partial visual loss -*pain-glaucoma acute* - redness, severe eye pain, sudden decrease vision and cloudy -*pain- periorbital –Cellulitis,* fever, eye swell and tender to touch	**Inflammation-**check for lice eggs-fresh white cabbage juice with a tiny amount of honey -compress -eye bright, or chickweed tea or witch hazel or tansy compress, noni -external eyewash- eyebright+ goldenseal+ fennel-strain in cloth -internal- eyebright+ bayberry+ red raspberry leaf +goldenseal+ cayenne

EYE DEFICIENCY SYMPTOMS

EFA =(essential fatty acids)

Bitot's spots-foamy patches on conjunctiva-Vitamin A

Blood shot -Boric acid for fungus infection, blue light

Blurred vision -Vitamin B 2, B6 pantothenic acid

Bulging eye -Vitamin E, nicitinamide, iodine (see thyroid)

Cataracts (lenses becomes opaque) -Vitamins B2, c, e antioxidants (avoid lactose)

Color-blindness -Vitamin A

Conjunctivitis -Vitamin a, B2, C (B6, zinc)

Cross-eyes -Vitamin E, C, B1 (allergic testing)

Dark spots in front of eyes -Vitamins B6, C, zinc (liver problems)

Dim vision (amblyopia) -Vitamin B1, B2, C, B12 (allergic testing)

Dry, hard eyeballs (exophthalmia) Vitamin A

Farsightedness (hyperopia) Magnesium, potassium, MSM

Glaucoma -Magnesium, vitamin C (B2, B1, salt)

Hemorrhaging in back of eyes (retinitis) Vitamin B6, zinc, bioflavonoids (also magnesium, vitamin C, B2, B12, E, pantothenate)

Infected, ulcerating eyes (keratomalacia) Vitamin A (vitamins C,B2, B6, zinc, blue light, boric acid)

Itching, burning, watery, sandy eyes Vitamin b2

Macular degeneration -Vitamin A, B2, B6, magnesium, zinc, antioxidants, bioflavonoids, esp. Lutein & zeaxanthin, gingko bilboa, bilberry, eyebright, MSM, EFA

Near-sightedness (myopia) Chromium, vitamins C, E, D, calcium (proteins, avoid sugars)

Night blindness (nyctalopia) Vitamins A (B6, B2, C, zinc)

Red blood vessels in the sclera Vitamin B2

Retinal detachment -Zinc, vitamins B6, B2, C, E, A

Sensitive eyes, fear of strong light (photophobia) Vitamins B2, A

Tics of eyelids- Magnesium, vitamins B2, B6, zinc

-apply lotion of eyebright or strained chickweed tea

-Light-weight Fomentations for 15 minutes, every 2 hours; frequently renewed cooling compress during intervals between

Inflammations of eyeball—a fomentation covering the eye (while the eye is closed) and extending to the forehead, for 15-20 minutes or until the skin is well-reddened. Repeat as often as necessary, to relieve pain. Employ the frequently renewed (5-15 minutes at 60^0 f.) Heating compress during the intervals between hot applications.

Night blindness-vitamin A (50,000 units daily) and 15-50 mg of zinc. -proven to improve night vision

Take 15-20 mg daily -bilberry extract capsules-pcos from grape seed or white pine (100mg 3x daily) -coq10 (60mg 3x daily -revulsive compress- warm compress longer than cold

Pale lid inside, - see anemia

Photophobia= light sensitive: -check for glaucoma- child who suddenly has that problem = early symptoms of measles

-vitamin A, carotene, yellow vegetables, carrots• take 50,000 units of vitamin a daily for a short time

Eyeball protruding out-see hyperthyroidism

Pigmented ring at the outer margin of the cornea of the eye- Wilson's disease

Puffy eyes: ice compress *borage wash

Red eyes- get more rest at night; lay a cool, wet washcloth over your closed eye. Eyebright, fennel, and cornflower. -vitamin-a, b2, b6 -cool wet cloth on

Soreness in eyeball with fever and face congestion-see dengue-white cabbage juice with a tiny honey

Sty -vitamin A; cleanse, Partially hot compress, alternated with cold, drink 3 cups of goldenseal tea or eyebright fennel or myrrh may be substituted. Tansy compress -raw potatoes poultice -3 cups goldenseal or eyebright tea or fennel or myrrh tea-apply concentrated thyme tea directly to the sty -drink Echinacea

Blurred vision; -eat dried unripe raspberries

Chalazon-swelling and pain disappear and leaves a pea like nodule on eyelid (usually due to a nutritional deficiency) -vitamin-a (beta carotene)- 50,000units for many days-drink carrot juice, eat green and yellow vegetables

-poultice od 3 % boric acid to closed lid-

-Take vitamin A (at least 50,000 units per day, as beta carotene, for a number of days. Also take zinc (50 mg, 3 times a day).

Color blindness -vitamin -A 5000iu daily and 25,000 iu of carotene take 50,000 units of vitamin a daily.

Child suddenly has sensitivity to light= early symptom of measles

Conjunctivitis (pink eye)

-mix 1/2 tsp fresh lemon + 4 oz. Distilled water drop in eye and cover eyearea with slice of onion that has been warmed apply bandage andon 5-8 hours (also decrease pressure in some eye)

-cucumber slicesover eye. Apply warm poultices of 3% boric acid on the closed lid.

-*During the day,* slurry charcoal water can be applied: Add ¼ tsp. Salt and 1 tsp. Powdered charcoal to a cup of water, boil, let cool, and strain through several layers of cloth. With a dropper, put 4-5 drops of the clear fluid on the affected eye every 2 hours.

-Ice-cold compresses can be laid on the eye during the acute stage. For half an hour, apply a wrung-out washcloth to the eye; change it every 2-3 minutes. Stop for 30-60 minutes, and then repeat for another 30 minutes.

- Hot and cold applications can be applied every 4 hours. But the water should never be too hot

Dark /red circles= body diseased-chamomile tea bags on closed eye

Crossed eyes: check for brain tumor **Dimness of eyes**: - add thyme to food angelica (do not use if pregnant)-addthyme to food

Dry tear ducts-vitamin-A, flaxseed, calcium, mg, bathe eye with aloe Vera juice, b-complex vit

-chamomile tea compress -swallow chopped garlic -take vitamin-a-swallow lots of raw garlic

Thinning eye lashes:-vit-a, b2, niacin -brewer's yeast 2 tbsp. Daily

-vitamin-e applied to eyelashes at night will thicken them (put it on gently)

Tunnel vision:- research shows bilberry and gingko bilboa both reduce this disease

-take- vitamin-A 15,000units daily (10,000units during pregnancy) -flaxseed oil 2 tbs. Daily -coenzyme q10 60mg 4x daily-pcos from grape seed or white pine 100mg 3x daily-taurine 500mg daily -zinc 20mg daily

Twitching eyelids: elder tea*

Ulcerated eye and lid caused by a virus, large doses of vitamin c (2,000 mg, 3 times a day). Apply warm yellow dock tea, in a poultice, to the eyelid. You can also drink it. Yellow dock tea poultice and drink

Visual loss progressive: vitamin-C, E, selenium, zinc, bilberry and lutein, taurine sublingually

Weak eyes: drink strong borage tea

Yellow eyes (icterus; jaundice) ultraviolet light exposure, Also obtain vitamins c, a, and e. Need liver cleanse

-*herbs*; combine the following- eyebright, blueberry leaves, lutein, goldenseal, bayberry, cayenne, bilberry, raspberry, chaparral tea, bilberry, dandelion, Norway kelp or nova scotia dulse

Herbal-a=acute; sa=subacute; c=chronic; d=degenerative

A(*conjunctivitis*) myrrh, eyebright, comfrey

Sa- (*sore, bloodshot*) goldenseal, raspberry, yarrow

C-(*night blindness, weak* tired) dandelion (fresh flowers), parsley, eyebright, yucca

D-(*cataract, glaucoma*) chaparral, eyebright, capsicum, mullein

Herbs -gingko bilboa, bilberry, eyebright, Essential fatty acids, golden seal, and red raspberry teas all help the eyes. Eyebright

+ b2,and zinc, vitamin A (50,000 units daily)- lack of it causes small openings to close down. -Essential fatty acids in your diet, calcium.

Infected:1/2 tsp salt to 8 oz. Water apply as eyewash -wash eyes with goldenseal root tea (do not use large amounts if pregnant) -charcoal poultice

-*cayenne restores eyesight* in some take 3x daily x months

-*wheat grass juice eye drop in eye*- itching and eye-strain

-*Swedish bitters*- spots, cataract, inflamed, detached retina, going blind, compress to eyes daily for 1 hour

Diet- selenium, and zinc. Eat greens every day. Nicotine, sugar, and caffeine all weaken the eyes.

FAINTING	
Open mouth and put 1 tbs. Swedish bitters in mouth or ½ tsp. Cayenne in mouth **Pound lightly on the back** between the shoulders/ **cold water to the face** **Frequent fainting spell-**teas- mint ,rue, catnip, mistletoe, rosemary, and a small amount of cayenne **Antispasmodic tincture-** 8 drops on the back tongue	**Hydrotherapy:-**alternate hot and cold compress over the spine-percussion of chest withhands/ or end of a towel dipped in cold water **Heat to neck and short cold application to chest and face** **Use your fist to pound slightly** on the back between the shoulders to stimulate the heart
FATIGUE	
Chronic fatigue- check for parasites-check for thiamine, calcium, potassium, vitamin B6+ C-deficiency -silver biotics-cleanse system-85% raw diet-green drink- 3 enemas daily for 7 days **Barley green and wheat grass are** *known to cure fatigue* **Supplement:-**potassium, iron, magnesium -take whole food vitamin supplements (especially b-complex vitamins -l-tyrosine 500 mg- overcomes fatigue, lemon water	**Herbs:-**Siberian / American ginseng, ginkgo - gotu kola, Jamaican sarsaparilla, ephedra, pasque flower, ginger, licorice-lemon balm, goldenseal Echinacea, Swedish bitters- take a sip and put on temples and around eyes **Hydrotherapy:-** hot tub bath-see alternate hot and cold shower -cold mitten friction
FEVER	
Fevers of 99° up to 102° = viral infection and minor inflammatory and bacterial diseases. Fevers above 104° usually reflect a bacterial infection such as *strep.* Or *staph.* **Fevers in children:**do not give aspirin-may cause death -hot sweat bath until sweating begins. -ages three months to three years, sit them hot tub for three minutes, with mother's arm submerged in the hot water for entire duration of bath, if child stand them up, *give a cold mitten friction,* followed by an ice cold water pour to whole body; rub dry and put to bed. **Child refusing to drink water-** put him in tub-body will absorb + catnip enema—will hydrate the child **1st sign**-garlic, ginger, cayenne, Echinacea-<u>cut a grape fruit</u>- expose the white covering-discard yellow cover cut in quarters put in boiling water	*Hydrotherapy-* see fomentation -see wet sheet pack (cooling stage) -early stage- skin hot, wet sheet pack(heating stage) -full body pack-neutral bath, wet sheet pack,cold mitten friction-steam bath,/ fever bath, salt bath, salt rub (2 treatments daily) *-ice packs on the forehead, running cool water over the wrists, cool baths and Wet compresses* ***Apple cider vinegar. Sponge.*** Then you simply give the person *a cool catnip* -cold garlic /catnip enema **Catnip tea enema** **Place 1/2 of an onion** underneath each feet and place sock on **If the fever gets too high** (above 102° F. In adults or 103° F. In children), immerse the body in tepid water to lower the temperature **Diet-**grapefruit, lemon juice, barley water, cayenne, carrot- beet- cucumber juice**,** barley water, cooked rice with lots of water

seeds and all - with anentire full bulb of <u>garlic</u> (crushed) drink **Vitamin C and lemon juice**	**Take 1 tbs. Swedish bitters,** noni, **white willow**= similar to aspirin
FIBROIDS in uterus	
Avoid supplements that contain PABA or large amounts of folic acid.**Formula**-Chaste tree, 1T in 1 quart water. Simmer 25 minutes. Drink daily until fibroids shrink. Use a fat-free diet. Take hot for bleeding after delivery. Use 1 tsp. To 1 C. Boiling water and cold sitz baths for a total of 30 minutes, alternating every five minutes of hot with one minute of cold, about 65-75°. **-disappear with- Echinacea + red root** Castor oil pack two to four times a week **Herbal suppository** use powdered herbs mixed with cocoa butter. Use red raspberry and equal quantities of wild yam pulverized in a blender or seed mill and mixed with melted cocoa butter (coconut oil) until you have a thin paste. Cool the mixture in the refrigerator. Use one tablespoon-size portion and roll into suppository size bars. Flatten slightly and cool in refrigerator before inserting. Use one nightly.	**Treatment Program:** Garlic (capsules): Take 2 twice a day for six weeks. You may later cut down to once a day after the six weeks. -Cayenne pepper mixed with goldenseal: 2 capsules twice a day. Echinacea tea: Mix at the rate of one teaspoon per cup. Drink one cup twice a day. -Use two tablespoons of liquid chlorophyll, unflavored (which contains iodine) **Douche**-One teaspoon of liquid dulse Lie in the knee-chest position or on one side with hips elevated on a pillow, and inject the liquid with a bulb syringe into the vagina as a retention douche. The next Night lie on the other side and have the retention douche. Do the douches every night and stay in the same position as long as possible before moving. In two to three fibroids will begin shrinking

GALLBLADDER

Herbal-a=acute; sa=subacute; c=chronic; d=degenerative

A-(inflammation) goldenseal, chaparral, cayenne, flaxseed

Sa-(sluggish) cayenne, goldenseal, mandrake, sanicle

C-(gallstones) flaxseed, olive oil, buchu, beet

D-(degenerative stage) Echinacea, goldenseal, chaparral

Diet- stop eating at attack-drink

Distilledwater fast for 2-3 days until the acute condition is past. Then go on juices for several more days. Apple, Pear juice, and beet juice best. Then add solid food, such as shredded raw beets with fresh lemon juice, olive oil, and freshly blended, uncooked applesauce. Pear. Oil is necessary in the diet. Avoid all meat, grease, processed fats and oils (including butter).

Gallbladder flush-4oz orange juice +4 oz. Lemon juice+ 5 Tbsp. Olive oil +5 cloves of garlic, fresh ginger, 15 oz. Water, pinch cayenne

Gallstones (bloating gas, discomfort, indigestion after heavy meals of rich, fatty food, may have constant pain below breastbone that shoots in right or left shoulder area and radiates to the back- pain may last 30 minutes to hours, chills ,fever-2 tbsp.)

Hydrotherapy- To relieve pain, give a 15 minutes hot fomentation over the gallbladder area, followed by an ice rub. Repeat the process 3 times.

-hot colonic or hot enema, every 2 hours; hot full bath.

-hot castor pack

-give liver flush

-*attack:*-peppermint, spearmint, catnip, cardamom-make tea drink-1st apply calendula ointment then moisture a piece of cotton ball with Swedish bitters put on area then cover with plastic- bandage with cloth and take 1 tbs. Internally- 3x daily-lecithin - catnip tea

-*Taking 2 tbsp. Of lecithin* each day immediately results in increased phospholipid concentration in the bile

-*dissolve it* :chamomile, dandelion tea- help dissolves ,lemon

Failure of gallbladder:4 oz. Beet juice 3x daily- will usually response in 24 hours and take a coffee enema (see cleanse)-1/2 cups lemon juice blended with 1/2 olive oil(lay on right side for 30 minutes)-to avoid vomit suck on lemon take 1 hour after enema and take herbal laxative

GANGRENE

Take a total body cleanser+ supplements (vitamin C, A, E cayenne)

Pour the sugar right on the wound. Keep putting sugar on the wound until it stops dissolving then it is ready to use your golden seal, your myrrh. If a sore is infected with germs, do not put goldenseal on top of it that will not help it .wrap this with Saran wrap.

1/4 ld. Charcoal + 1oz. Cayenne or smartweed-steep x 20 minutes mix with 2ld. Whole wheat flour put on gauze and cover area-may add garlic to the poultice -marshmallow root tea packs to area

When pus is oozing, dab warm hydrogen peroxide on, and wipe off carefully.

If **the gangrene** severe-one ounce iodine and mix it into a pound of sugar. Apply this on the wound.	**Apply cool leg baths or cool whole baths**. Chaparral tea or apple cider vinegar can be added to the water, to help disinfect it (about 1 tbsp. Per quart). -alternate hot and cold foot baths or fomentation packs, to improve blood flow.

GAS IN THE STOMACH

Check for iron deficiency, see stomach for achlorhydria - insufficient stomach acid. Causes belching, bloating, burping **Flatulence**: check for iron deficiency -check for parasites *Diet*-chew slowly- don't talk while chewing -walk after meals (leisure stroll)-low fat diet -avoid carbohydrate drink-chewing gum -do not postpone bowel movements -avoid gas forming foods (beans, soy beans, prune juice, lima beans, broccoli, cauliflower, peas, celery, corn, apples, Brussels sprouts, kohlrabi, radishes, raisins, cucumber, onions, cabbage, bananas, apple juice,-legumes some, some fruits and some grains are gas forming) -**GI detox:** 2 parts charcoal, 3 parts bentonite clay, 7 parts psyllium seed powder, 2 part marshmallow root powder, 1 part fennel powder stir 1 tbs. Into 1 glass of water or juice. Drink immediately. Do this 2-3x daily ½ hour before meals	**Comfrey fomentation**- blend fresh comfrey and hot water in the blender- soak a handful in the solution. Wring out, fold once and place over the lower abdomen for 30 minutes. Use a hot fomentation over the top to keep it warm **Heating** trunk and hips are wrapped, the extremities excluded. A hot foot bath is given simultaneously. **Formula-** = part peppermint herb, Senna leaves, coriander seed, anise seed and caraway seed- (seeds should be powdered and mixed- take one tsp in a cup of boil h2o- let stand x10 min. Take 2-3x daily **Herbs :** 2 tsp. Of vinegar in a glass of water ,*take Swedish bitters-charcoal-* no chewing gum -1tsp of anise seed + 1 part honey mix in 1 glass of water-boil x 10 minutes-let cool-strain take 1-2 tbs. Daily **Gastric faulty stomach:** ginger root *Take*-hot enema

GASTRITIS

Gastritis may be acute or chronic. Chronic gastritis leads to atrophy of the stomach, with slow decreased acid and pepsin. This causes poor digestion, malabsorption of vitamin b-12 (pernicious anemia), and stomach cancer **Aloe Vera:** -aloe Vera is used for gastrointestinal problems **Persistent stomach problems**-check for helicobacter -treat with goldenseal, Echinacea, grapefruit seed extract, and garlic for one month.(bring one quart of water to a boil, when simmering gently add one slightly rounded tablespoon of	**Vomiting**-ice bag to epigastrium -hot and cold compress over the stomach -ice to spine opposite the stomach **Gastric acid over-production**, charcoal powder, one tablespoonful four times daily **Gastrointestinal conditions:-**diarrhea, nausea, and vomiting-hot sweat bath as described under "common cold."-charcoal tablets, four to eight every four hours for two to three doses. Bland diet scraped fresh apple. Carob powder made to a paste with water, one to two tablespoons. Catnip tea.

goldenseal powder and one heaping tablespoon of Echinacea.) Gently simmer for 20 minutes, strain, and drink throughout each day for 30 days. To each cup of tea, add 8- to 10 drops of grapefruit seed extract . If that much *grapefruit seed extract* causes a stomachache, drop the dosage to four to six drops. Eat a whole globe of *garlic* microwaved for 1 minute and 10-15 seconds at each meal. A globe of garlic contains 12-15 cloves.	**Herbal-**calendula tea -chamomile, ginger, turmeric, marshmallow or slippery elm -take mustard seed the first day and increase by 1 seed succeeding morning for 20 days the decrease seeds by 1 every morning for 20 days (do not take treatment at night) **Hydrotherapy-**local inflammation- fomentations over stomach and bowels x 15 minutes every 2hours-during intervals - heating compress at 60f. Changing every 30 minutes-hot foot bath: hot leg packs

GASTROENTERITIS(stomach flu)

Symptoms =diarrhea, nausea, vomiting, abdominal. Pain, loss appetite-last 24-72 hours -check for underlying problems- anemia, b12 deficiency, bacterial, acid problems **Catnip-**mix 1 tsp. Of catnip tea leaves in a cup of water, steep for 15 minutes, and drink while warm. **Eat:-**fast for a few days, cooked rice, plain cooked potatoes. Cooked carrotsbananas, applesauce **Formula:-**mix 1 oz. Each of flaxseed, slippery elm, boneset and a stick of licorice-simmer x 20 minutes-in 1 qt. Water- strain- add 1 pt. Apple cider vinegarand sweeten-keep cool-give 1-2 tbs. 2-3 x daily	**Herbs:-** catnip tea- amaranth* -Swedish bitters **Diet-**When vomiting and diarrhea cease, give small amounts of non-irritating food, such as cooked carrots, bananas, or apple sauce cooked rice, plain cooked potatoes,.Avoid processed and greasy foods; avoid milk and high-roughage foods. **If fluids cannot be kept down**, give small saline enemas. Using 1 level tsp. Of salt per pint of water, inject 1-2 oz. Of the solution into the rectum (using a small rubber bulb syringe). Then hold the buttocks together for several minutes. Do this every 1-2 hours until improvement is seen, and he is able to take fluids

GLANDS

Swollen Gland +Undescended +lymphatic-Testicle: three parts mullein and one part lobelia herb and use as a fomentation over swollen or malfunctioning glands. Leave on all night (covering fomentation with plastic), six days a week until relief is obtained. Do external fomentation, drink a cup of this tea two or three times in a day or take two of the capsules or tablets with a cup of steam-distilled water. *Diet-*-drink 2-3 qt. Water daily -5- 14 days fruit juice fast-high potassium diet (potatoes, onions, carrots, banana) **Supplement:**vit- b complex, a (over 19 glands needs vitamin-a),c, zinc supplement	**Apply to liver-** lymphatic flow and liver activity. Blend 1 clean whole lemon (pulp, rind, seeds, and all) 1 tablespoon of extra virgin olive oil+1 ½ cups of distilled water 4 rounded tablespoons of frozen orange juice concentrate 2-3 qt. Water **Poultice:** carrot, castor oil packs, lavender lotion/ water bruised parsley -comfrey/, plantain/, apple cider vinegar and witch hazel-use one or more-poultice; carrot/ castor oil packs/ lavender lotion or lavender water/ parsley tea Pregnancy- they also apply 2 parts turmeric and 1 part salt to area

Formula: 1part=1tbs.(mix the following take 6 capsules 2x daily)gentian 3 part ,yellow dock 1 part bayberry bark 1 part, prickly ash 1 part, golden seal1 part , st. John's wort 1 part

Irish moss 1 part ,blue vervain 1 part, comfrey 2 part, mandrake 1 part milk thistle 2 part , pau d'arco 3 part

Herbs: -garlic enema (3x daily)-take a cleanser 5x daily -goldenseal(2 cap 2x daily) -echinacea (10 cap daily) -pau d'arco (10 cap daily) -garlic (blend 5 bulbs with little water- take 1 tsp 5x daily)

Daily-salt glow-steam bath daily 1x for 10 days or fever bath daily x 10 days then 3x weekly alternate with fever bath

See castor oil packs (in cleanse section)(usually for one hour daily)

Take ginger- 2oz. Daily x 30+ days also apply 2 parts turmeric + 1 part salt to area pineapple compound 400-500mg 3x daily

Fomentation: of decoction of rue

A day)

Compress: 2oz. Mullein+ 1/2 oz. Lobelia+ 1tsp. Cayenne simmer in 2 qt. Apple cider vinegar – cover x 15 min. Strain and apply cool

-comfrey, plantain, apple cider vinegar, witch hazel,

Pituitary gland formula

All stages- ginseng, dong quai, gotu kola, safflower, kelp, damania

-formula- carrot leaf ,gotu kola for nourishment, ginkgo, mullein for cleansing, Oregon grape and lobelia as an overall catalyst for the formula.

GLAUCOMA

Symptoms: eye pain or discomfort especially in the morning, blurred vision, halos around sources of light, inability to adjust to darker conditions, peripheral (side vision) loss

Cause: increase ocular pressure**hydrotherapy- colon cleanse-hot _(not too hot)_**and cold to eye

-_hot compress for 9 minutes_ followed by cold for1 min. For 1 hour daily

-_take a hot foot bath_ (if not diabetic) every morning and every evening by all means,

-_application of hot_ compresses to the eyes for nine minutes, then exchange with one minute of cold. Repeat the process six times. Continue the treatment for a month or two, until improvement is obvious.

-_herbs_-gingko- 1tbs 3x daily, vitamin- a 15,000iu 3x daily, vitamin-c 5000 mg 3x daily- lemon juice 1 drop in each eye in a honey 1 drop in each eye in pm

Intense exercise for at least 15 minutes daily will drop the intraocular pressure by as much as five millimeters of mercury.

Poultice: -clay pack to closed eye -onion poultice to closed eye-lobelia and flax seed poultice and again at noon if possible.

At night one should put a very light pressure bandage on the eyes, about the equivalent of pressure from a folded wet washcloth laid on one eye when one is lying down,

Large doses of vitamin c are claimed to cure "open angle glaucoma." The patient as much as possible without getting diarrhea, in three daily doses

Coleus forskohlii **reduce** the pressure

Egg white to paper towel and apply to closed eye

GONORRHEA

Symptoms:-_women_- vaginal itching, frequent and painful urination and a cloudy vaginaldischarge. Inflammation of the pelvic area, abnormaluterine bleeding, rectal discharge,

-men-yellowish, pus-like urethral discharge-_both_

Hyacinth bean- leaves-infusion***

Drink 3 cups daily of: skullcap, hops, white oak bark, uvaursi, sage , poplar red carrot, + juniper -drink at least 3 cups slippery elm tea daily take 2 high enemas daily

sexes- very often (especially in women)-there is no symptoms

-often there are no symptoms for months- especially in women yet they are contagious

Hydrotherapy- pain: -warm sitz baths, 2-3 times daily -hot fomentation for pain to legs etc.

Take-acute cases: mix black willow, skullcap, + saw palmetto berries-steep a heaping tsp. In a cup boiling water x 1/2 hours -take 2 tbs. 6x daily+ take other herbs -in addition use herbs listed on syphilis also

Cleansing program of fruit juices take 2 high enemas daily

Supplements: -beta-carotene (150,000 iu. Daily) and 1/2 tsp. Vitamin-c powder, every hour to bowel tolerance, during the acute stage later reduce vit-c to 5,000mg daily, for 1 month

Wash sores: myrrh, goldenseal, witch hazel, chickweed, sorrel-tea of 1 part aloes and 2 parts goldenseal and myrrh

Female =douche- tea raspberry leaves and witch hazel leaves

Formula- burdock 2 part -cleaver 2 part -goldenseal 1 part -hops 2 part-parsley 2 part -juniper berries 2 part -squaw vine 1 part

GOUT

Mud packs, applied

Do not fast when you have gout ,

avoid cold baths of any kind

Least 2 quarts of water a day between gout attacks

Diet- cherries is very helpful.

Avoid Here are foods high in purines: (liver, brains, kidneys, heart, anchovies, sardines, meat extract, fish roes, herring, consommé, mussels, and sweet breads).

Avoid-excessive food yeast

At night- potatoes + onion poultice leave on all night7-8 nights in a row-charcoal poultice helpful -blended comfrey root or leaves and apply for pain

Charcoal. Take it by mouth (12-16 tablets daily)

Compress of comfrey root or leaves, blended with water, helps relieve gout pain. Apply for two hours or more, or overnight.

-apply tincture of lobelia, apple cider vinegar and honey

Make a paste with cayenne and wintergreen oil -hot fomentation- 15 minutes every 3 hours

Burdock will help clean uric acid deposits from the joints and other areas. Kelp, red clover, and yucca help eliminate uric acid and other toxins.

Yucca - eliminates uric acid

HAIR

Baldness and hair loss (Alopecia)

Adequate protein in the diet (especially vegetable seeds, such as sesame, pumpkin, sunflower, almonds), brewer's yeast and fresh brewer's yeast -Take a good supplement at least twice a day. Drink fresh vegetable juice at least once a day. Take vitamin A (50,000 units daily). B vitamins. Eat sea kelp or dulse. Biotin, inositol, niacin, vitamin E, and PABA are also important. Biotin up to 10,000 mg

Oat straw and horsetail tea. Rosemary , Sage is an astringent, Yarrow

-MSM, diatomaceous earth (1 tbs. Daily)

Dandruff- rub quince juice to scalp massage burdock root oil into scalp

-4 heaping tsp. Eucalyptus leaves to 1 qt. Boiling water cover and let steep for 1 hour-strain and pour in squeeze bottle and add 1 tbs. Apple cider vinegar- pour over head and let dry

Diet includes flaxseed oil, vitamins E and A, PABA, Folic acid, B$_6$, and zinc. **Oily skin**: squeeze the juice of 2 lemons into a pint of water and use it as a finishing rinse-or use an apple cider rinse massage and leave in for 5 minutes then rinse of

Dry hair: sesame seed oil / flaxseed oil to hair

-massage avocado to hair- mix 1 peeled avocado- + 1 tsp jojoba oil and wheat germ oil- after shampoo cover hair with plastic for 15-30 minutes- do weekly

Aloe - as shampoo and/or conditioner

Grey hair-to restore natural color to gray hair, the following vitamins have been reported to be successful for some people: paba (para-amino benzoic acid), pantothenic acid, folic acid, along with brewer's yeast, and blackstrap molasses. Also take a good multi-vitamin/mineral formula. Include some kelp or dulse in your diet.

Herbal-a=acute; sa=subacute; c=chronic; d=degenerative

A-(dandruff) nettle, burdock, sarsaparilla

Sa-(slow growing, dullness) sunflower seed, rosemary, kelp, cayenne, nettle (psoriasis) nettle, echinacea, sarsaparilla. (scrofula) bayberry root bark, cayenne, nettle

HEADACHE

Note: Anemia-if with fatigue, dizziness, shortness of breath on exertion-sudden severe headache- go to ER= aneurism-see Swedish bitters- apply to temple and take internally

-chronic- check for parasites, noni

Headache and migraines: lots of headaches comes from constipation- cleanse the colonpain tea- 1 tsp. White willow bark or wild lettuce- 1 cup boiling water- pour water over the herbs-steep 15- 20 minutes, strain and drink as often as needed

Migraine Headaches-(allergy= cause most of time)-butternut

Glass of cold water every 10

Minutes for 1 hour

Hydrotherapy-*hot mustard tub:* prepare bathtub with three to four inches of hot water. Add one tablespoon mustard.

Immerse forearms to elbows and feet and legs in the water. Maintain heat for twenty minutes.

Headaches: use 1 heaping teaspoonful of ground cayenne pepper (from the spice section of the-supermarket). Put in about 2 ounces of rubbing alcohol and shake vigorously 3 times a day for about 3 days. Let settle then, and he top.

Saline-put 2 drops into an ounce of normal saline (make it by putting a level tsp of salt into a pint of distilled water), and shake well. Put several drops of this mixture into the involved nostril, holding the head back. Opt. Use a nasal

Cayenne pepper extract for cluster Hydrotherapy-hot foot bath -ice compress- congested head-ice cap to head-congested head -hot pack to leg and hip-hot and cold head treatment -*cold spray*. Apply a cold spray to soles of feet for five seconds while a cold compress is applied to forehead.	sprayer, one spray is enough. It will burn! But wears off within a few minutes. Do this 6 times a day for 6 days.

HEART

CARDIAC ARREST-at first symptom:- you have 10 seconds before loss of consciousness- -*Immediately*-cough repeatedly andvery vigorously-take a deep breath before each cough- (the cough must be deep and prolonged)- -repeat a breath and a cough every 2 seconds without rest-this causes heart to receive oxygen and increase survival rate - *have arnica* with you at all time if you have risk -*preventive*-cayenne daily + put under tongue at 1st sign of arrest*squirt- cayenne (1tsp.) Water in the mouth +take arnica if available, see anti spasmodic tincture -cold bag (ice pack) over heart for 15 minutes -cold mitten friction every 2 hours- followed by a cold towel rub -hot enema- followed by cold-enema -hot blanket pack for 10 minutes **Cardiac arrest heart attach:**1/2 tsp *cayenne*pepper in 1 oz. Warm water - hold head back and swallow <u>avoid</u>-tip or side of tongue -unconscious- put cayenne pepper under tongue -*Myocardial infarction:* -vitamin C, e, selenium, HCL supplementsRebuilding afterward should include vitamin C to bowel tolerance, Vitamin B complex, A, E, Flaxseed oil , wheat germ oil , Lecithin Selenium, Brewer's yeast and chromium, pancreatic enzymes. Bran fiber Garlic, Alfalfa, Soy protein lowers blood cholesterol. Heart Tincture: 1-Use the above Cayenne Pepper Tincture Method with 3 parts - Hawthorn Berry, Flower & Leaf, 1 part - Red Clover Blossoms, 1 part - Garlic Bulb, 1 part - Cactus Grandiflorus Stem,	**Weak-irregular heart:**-formula- mix 1 tsp each- black cohosh, valerian, skullcap, lobelia + pinchof cayenne- add 1 tsp to 1 cup boiling water steep x 30 min. Take 4 cupsdaily / 1 swallow every 2 hours **Weak heart-** check for magnesium deficiencys-*trengthen heart*-skullcap, valerian, borage, tansy, **Weak heart:** - cold compress or ice bag over heart x 15 min. Every 2 hours. Cold mittenfiction every 2 hours -prolonged neutral baths -with ice bag over heartcold pail pour over back of head and back of spine after bath -cold compress or ice bag over the heart, alternate (hot then cold)applications to the spine, cold mitten friction, cold towel rub- repeating-treatment hourly if needed *Formula:*#1:-motherwort - 1 part -hawthorn -2 part -cayenne -1 part #2-tincture of fresh Hawthorne berry, leaf and flower, red clover blossoms, cactus grandiflorus stem/ flower, motherwort herb, garlic bulb, Jamaican ginseng root and cayenne (reduces blood pressure, blood fat, cholesterol, tones heart) -eat 3-6 cloves of garlic daily <u>Formula hawthorn berry heart syrup</u>-Dosages: one half teaspoon three times in a day.-Ingredients:Hawthorn berry syrup is made with hawthorn berry juice concentrate using grape brandy and glycerin as aids and preservatives. *Hawthorn berry in combination with cayenne will tone the heart and will help stimulate the heart to renew and rebuild.*- give four three times a day *I like to give hawthorn in capsules, and in tea.* With the capsules,-To make the tea, use one tablespoon powder in water. Drink this tea three

1 part - Motherwort, 1 part - Cayenne Pepper and 1 part - Ginger Root.
-Take 2-3 Dropperfuls - 3-4 times per Day, if needed.

Supplement:-coenzyme q10 -lecithin -red yeast rice extract - l- arginine-wheat germ oil- increase oxygen levels by 30% -pycnogenol-eat nova scotia dulse or Norwegian kelp- for trace minerals -selenium deficiency linked to heart disease- Avoid vitamin D. Cold-pressed flaxseed oil or wheat germ oil; also take selenium, vitamin E, 5-10 alfalfa tablets daily. And, if needed, obtain hcl. Take a 30-minute walk outside every day

Herbal for all heart problems:-hot cayenne 1/2 tsp- 1 tsp 3x daily -hawthorn extract ***lecithin, vitamin e*or caps 2x daily

A=acute; sa=subacute; c=chronic; d=degenerative

A-(high blood pressure) Hawthorne berries, mistletoe, cayenne

Sa- (weak, low blood pressure) angelica, borage, Hawthorne berries

C-(arteriosclerosis) fenugreek seed, kelp, pleurisy root, Hawthorne berries

D-(chronic heart failure) Hawthorne, cayenne, coriander

Hydrotherapy- do salt glow -daily skin brushing- do not do alt hot and cold shower-weak heart-**do not do neutral bath -do not do steam inhalation

Anticoagulant-natures instead of aspirin:-5 ounces of purple grape juice daily, -1 clove of garlic daily, 4-8 tablets daily-hawthorn berry tea- 4 cups daily -feverfew, gingko bilboa

Lily of the valley- _has action similar to digitalis_ -use with supervision*

*Palpitations:*Do not eat MSG, caffeine, sugar, or processed foods. Avoid food allergens. Obtain vitamins B1, B3, C, selenium, and potassium.

Pericarditis, endocarditis - ice bag over heart, cold compress over heart area (60f.) Change every 15 minutes, rub chest with dry flannel until chest is red

times a day. Cayenne. If you give ½ teaspoon under the tongue to someone who is having a heart attack, it will revive their heart in about 60 seconds.

Cardiotonic:cramberry-8oz. Juice 2xdaily

Edema-helps kidneys reduce edema-rosemary -*helps recovery-gingko

Cardiac arrhythmia Hypoglycemia can be a cause. Avoid food allergens and MSG. Add selenium, motherwort, chromium, magnesium, valerian, angelica, potassium, and coq10 to your diet. -selenium, chromium, mg, potassium, taurine, astralagus, valerian

Cardiomyopathy(keshan disease):-it is a selenium deficiency disease= know treatment

Congenital heart failure -supplements:-vitaminb1 , mg, selenium,- arginine (5.6-12.6g) daily -taurine(6g daily)- carnine (500mg 2-3x daily) -potassium (potatoes peeling soup) -coenzyme q10-magnesium (300mg daily) -selenium-hawthorn-(80-300mg 2x daily) or tincture (4-5ml 3x daily)

Congestive heart failure: Causes can include lung disease and high blood pressure. Obtain vitamin B1 and selenium.

Irregular heartbeat- check magnesium deficiency

Myocarditis: treatment - no ice bag over chest -see pericarditis for hydrotherapy-selenium supplements **post nervous heart:** check for anemia+ low stomach acid -b1, b12, iron

-formula- mix = part valerian root, lavender flowers, chamomile fennel-steep 2 tsp in 1/2 cup boiling- hot water take 1- 1 1/2 cups daily in mouthfuls*Nervous heart:* Causes can include anemia and low stomach acid. Obtain B1 and iron.

Palpitations:- vitamin -b1, b3,c selenium, potassium -check for iron deficiency -lemon water- wild cherry bark tea -lily of the valley, angelica, -blue cohosh, cayenne,goldenseal -wood betony, valerian, vervain-formula- tansy -1 tsp to 1 cup boiling water take 3-4cups daily*palpitation-* blue cohosh*,** black haw, check iron, calcium deficiency-

-to energize heart and maintain vital resistance- cold towel rub 2x daily, cold mitten friction -fever- prolonged neutral bath, neutral wet sheet - pain-fomentation for 1-3 minutes every 15 minutes during the interval Between **Tachycardia: (heart rate too fast)** Motherwort-powder-1Tbs.Hawthorn powder 1Tbs.-Cayenne-1Tbs. Mix all together these powdered herbs and make capsules. Take 2 capsules 3 times daily.*To slow heart rate*- vitamin-b1 *Slow- rate if have increase heart rate:*cayenne	

HEMOPHILIA

Cause: hereditary **Diet-**high in vitamin –K, alfalfa, broccoli, kale, all green leafy veg. Alfalfa, broccoli, egg yolks, Green drinks	**Vitamin-t proven to combat this** **Supplement:** vitamin. K 300mg daily, b- complex vitamin, niacin, vitamin-c 3000 mg daily,-calcium- 1500mg daily, magnesium- 1000mg daily

HEMORRHOIDS

Squeeze *lemon juice* in rectum - make alum tea and inject several x daily * **Apply**-ginger tea or yarrow *extract*-goldenseal / ginger / yarrow tea-plantain, Apply cold witch hazel tea -Cranberry poultices-Blend a handful, wraps a tablespoonful in cloth, and lay against the area. Change an hour later, and repeat as needed -Dab lecithin on the area, -An ice pack to that area -Peel a garlic bulb and scrape it, to get the juice, to flow. Then insert it. It will be expelled the next day during elimination. Do this 3 times a week. -Applications of white oak bark tea or witch hazel will, **Bleeding hemorrhoids:** lyre leaves, sage, aloe suppository-suppository with witch hazel	**Sitz baths** (hot) 100 degrees for 10-20 minutes add a cup of witch hazel • *In severe cases, take an alternating hot and cold sitz* (sitting) bath. **Suppository:** *aloe*- cut 2 ½ inch inside in suppository shape and freeze- 3x daily-cocoa butter (melted)2 oz. + stir in 2 tbsp. Finely powdered (witch hazel, bayberry, yellow dock mold into suppository and freeze -cut up *white potatoes* as a suppository- put between both cheeks or inside -*formula*: glycerin/ cucumber + goldenseal 2 part+ bayberry 2 part+ chickweed 2 partwitch hazel 2 part +catnip 1/4 part (mix and refrigerate)

HEPATITIS

Research show bioflavonoids curesymptoms— weakness, nausea, headache, vomiting, fever, joint stiffness and pains, muscle aches, loss of appetite, drowsiness, dark urine, abdominal discomfort, diarrhea, constipation, light-colored stools, and often jaundice. Skin rashes and itching may also occur	**Hydrotherapy-**hot fomentation to liver x15 minutes then alternate with cold for 4 minutes daily-strengthens the liver- fever bath - increase body temperature 102-104 x20 min. Keep head cool do x 10-15 days -castor oil pack over liver for discomfort-burdock leaf pack over inflamed liver

Hepatitis A (infectious hepatitis): Transmitted by contaminated water, milk, or food, it has an incubation period of 15-45 days. The contagion is highest just before illness begins, so food workers can transmit the disease. Hepatitis A is contagious from 2 weeks to 1 week before the illness starts. It is easily spread by person-to-person contact and through contact with food, clothing, linens, etc. It can be transmitted from animals. Eating shellfish

Hepatitis B (serum hepatitis): infected blood (contaminated needles, syringes, blood transfusions) and sexual contact. It has an incubation period of 28-160 days (2-6 months), and recovery may require 6 months.

Hepatitis C: Contracted in the same manner as HIV and hepatitis B, hepatitis C may take 6 months to produce symptoms, yet all that time it can be spread from one person to another. It accounts for 90-95% of all hepatitis transmitted by blood donations.

Hepatitis E, hepatitis non-A, and hepatitis non-B contracted from drinking sewage-contaminated water.

-strong peppermint tea with a pinch of cayenne as a poultice over liver

Other treatments: take cleanser -chlorophyll enemas 3x weekly use 1 pt. And retain for 15 minutes-castor oil pack over liver- keep warm – **herbs**-burdock leaf pack over liver silymarin and ginkgo. Take the silymarin, derived from the milk thistle, one cup oftea or two capsules three or four times a day.

Vitamins B₁₂ and C are important CHARCOAL-charcoal compresses and charcoal by mouth (one tablespoon three to four timesdaily) as well as wheat bran by mouth (one tablespoon with each meal). –

Japanese clinicians have used glycyrrhizin, an extract of licorice-astragals root, , and turmeric

Jaundice produces itching it can be relieved by giving guar gum.

Grapefruit seed extract(10 drops 3x daily) for 1 month in juice

CHARCOAL-charcoal compresses and charcoal by mouth (one tablespoon three to four timesdaily) as well as wheat bran by mouth (one tablespoon with each meal) can reducethe amount of bile salts and the degree of jaundice.

HERNIA

Symptoms—heartburn and belching. There may be difficulty in swallowing. Material from the stomach may suddenly return into the throat or mouth, causing a burning sensation. It may feel as if there is a lump in the throat, or that food is sticking at a point in the throat. Sometimes bloody mucous is coughed up.

Check copper deficiency

If the hernia ring is larger than your finger tip, surgery is needed, to correct

Elevation of the head of the bed on 8-10 inch blocks may help

Wear a truss

Hernia in a child is less serious, and the opening may repair itself if the protruding bowel loop is pushed back and held in place by a firm band or adhesive strap for a few months.

Hernia in a child-three time daily- remove wool ball -make sure skin is pushed down firmly - at that time rub the hernia ring in a circular motion x several minutes-be patient - takes several months or weeks *hiatal hernia*-poultice- comfrey leaves, bistort root, and giant Solomon's seal root-renew every 12hours

-shave grass tea compress-.do poultice at night and compress during the day

Strong tea of white oak bark- one cup to 1 qt. Water- boil x 2 min- let stand x 2 hours –strain and add 1 tsp alum powder- fold piece of cloth to area soaked in tea and cover with plastic- repeat 4x daily x 1 months

HERPES (type II) venereal	
Symptoms:-itching, burning in the genital area, discomfort during urination, a watery vaginal orurethral discharge, weeping fluid like eruptions on vagina or penis-can be passed to baby during childbirth **Black walnut hull tincture** **Cures it** **Apply-**DMSO to area ,t-tree oil **Internally/ externally: -** black walnut/ goldenseal extract or cayenne and red clover	**Formula:** powdered herbs- 25% each echenesea and chaparrel-12% each sarsaparilla, oregano grape root -10% poria cocos-8% each licorice, and ginger -put in 00 caps. -take -2 caps each -3-4 x daily x 3 months **Pain and inflammatory**: -ice to area **Hydrotherapy:** -fever therapy , hot bath -expose sunlight to lesions **herbs**: goldenseal, Echinacea, myrrh, aloe Vera, burdock peppermint oil to genital
HICCUP	
Hiccups which will not stop, go on a 3 day complete fast. **Fill a glass of water and place a metal object** such as a spoon / knife and sip slowly holding part of the metal against your temple with bottom part in water **Hot bath** for 15 minutes. **Ice bag to** the pit of the stomach.	*Take 1 tsp. Of fructose the result is immediate* if hiccups will not stop- do a 3 day juice fast **Swallow a teaspoonful of sugar** **Put ice on the neck.** Drink catnip tea.Chew and swallow ice for 10-15 minutes. **Fresh orange juice-**Drink a half glassful
HIGH BLOOD PRESSURE	
For low blood pressure see hypotension **Barley green known to cure** **Herbal-**cayenne 1 caps 3x daily -1 oz. Watermelon seed crushed- pour on 1 cup boil water- strain- take 1c before meals -Hawthorn berry in combination with cayenne **Blend turnip** and drink the water **Blend garlic** 3 cloves with 1 eggplant (cut in small pieces)- soak overnight in distilled or mineral water and drink- ¼ cups 3x daily	**Submerge feet in garlic** water while taking steam bath **Diet-juice fast for 3-5 days-** -*eat raw garlic and onions* Fruit and rice diet- alone, for 1-2 weeks **Fruit and rice, alone, for 1-2 weeks.** **Hydrotherapy-**wet sheet pack -nightly for 1 week Epson salt soak with 2 1/2 ld.in bath - **Formula:**1 cut up eggplant 1 qt. Distilled water+2 cloves of garlic +burdock 1/2 tsp powder / 1 tbsp. Leaves leave in jar overnight(take 3-4 oz. 3x daily)
HODGKIN'S	
Symptoms—fatigue, itching, fever, general sickish feeling, night sweats, weakness, weight loss, enlargement of lymph nodes and spleen which is generally not painful. **Cause:**-lymphatic organs (spleen, nodes, tonsils, appendix)- when either of these areremoved or become clogged- too much waste matter id=s being channeledthrough- trouble occurs	**Fever bath** 3x weekly, salt glow, steam baths, hot and cold water treatments **Enema:** black strap molasses 2x daily (use 1 tbsp. Of black strap molasses in 1 pt.h2o) . Keep the bowels open. Do not strain at the stool, for this could injure a temporarily enlarged spleen. **Take vitamin- k** 2x daily- 4 drops of iodine (see weed) 2x daily

Go on a vegetable juice fast for 2-3 days, then eat nourishing food, and fast again every few days. **Hydrotherapy**-steam baths, salt glows, and hot and cold water treatments will invigorate the body	**Hodgkin's lymphoma**- a. Echinacea burdock, pau d'arco, red clover, white oak bark, plantain, vervain, yarrow **Herbs** include Echinacea, burdock, pau d'arco, and red clover. Other herbs include white oak bark, plantain, vervain, and yarrow **Black strap molasses 2x** daily (use 1 tbsp. Of black strap molasses in 1 pt. Water enema **Poultice:** clay over swollen Glands, hot castor oil, hot charcoal +flaxseed poultice over swollen glands, do mud bath weekly
## HYPOGLYCEMIA (low blood sugar)	
Check-milk allergy **Herbs:** licorice, bilberry, wild yam, cedar berries, spirulina tabs, milk thistle, ginger**,** dandelion coffee, blueberry leaf tea, chickpea roasted (coffee) lecithin – 2 tbs. Daily**.** Huckleberry tea	**Supplement:** vitamin-c, e magnesium, chromium, potassium, zinc **Formula**: licorice root powder- approximately 3-7 capsules daily, agar agar- 1 tbs. Daily in juice. Vitamin-b complex 20-300 mcg daily, niacin 250 mg daily
## HYPOTENSION(low blood pressure)	
Check magnesium deficiency-You may want to do the morning temperature test to determine whether you are hypothyroid **Supplement:** vitamin-c (1000- 3000mg) daily, vitamin-e (100iu gradually increase to 600 iu.)- Take vitamin C, to bowel tolerance, and eight glasses of water each day. Obtain adequate rest at night.	**Russian steam bath** **Herbs:** dandelion greens, dandelion tea, ginger root, skullcap with a pinch ofcayenne, ginger teas ,ginseng, sage, rosemary, thyme, winter savory,hawthorn, lily of the valley, camphor tree, cayenne 1 capsules 3x daily **Eat garlic**-beet juice- 6 oz. Glass daily-greens

IMMUNE

SEE CASTOR OIL PACK IN CLEANSE SECTION

Sugar decreases immune system by 50%

Increase the immune system:-fasting -hot and cold contrast shower- stimulates bone toproduce stem cells (hot x 6 minutes, cold x 1 minutes) do 2x daily for 3 days weekly -3cycles each time

Herbs: astralagus, Echinacea, lomatium- osha, cat's claw, paud'arco ,spirulina, chaparral, dandelion, red clover, and kelp.

-DHEA- detox**,** quince, blue false indigo, garlic, dandelion, red clover, kelp, alfalfateas (antimicrobial)—(these teas should be taken continuously by those having a serious chronic disease).

-Echinacea and chaparral: put one heaping tablespoon of Echinacea in one quart of boiling water and boil gently for 30 minutes. Turn the flame off and add 2 tablespoons of chaparral. Let this mixture steep for 15 minutes. Drink one cup first thing in the morning and finish the remainder of the quart throughout the day. Do this daily

(b) *pau d'arco, blue violet and red clover:* add 3 tablespoons of pau d'arco to one quart of boiling water and boil gently for 15 minutes. Turn flame off, add 2 tablespoons of blue violet and 2 tablespoons of red clover to the pau d'arco and let the mixture steep for 15 minutes.

Green papaya- protects immune system

Swedish bitters+ noni- immune system booster**,** silver biotic **selenium and vitamin-e** , zinc a must-

Formula:blend-1/2 grapefruit-1 orange-1 lemon -1/2 medium onion -2-4 garlic cloves peeled-3-4 drops peppermint oil -1/4 cup water (take 2-4 tbsp. As often as needed)

Rocket fuel: blend together-1- medium onion +1-2 tbsp. Powdered ginger (or 1 1/2 piece) + 6-8 lemon +5 garlic cloves + pinch cayenne honey to taste +horse radish for congestion

-cut 3 large onions +/ 3 large bulbs of garlic into 1 ½ qt. Water- cook till tender, strain- drink 1 cup every 30 minutes (add cayenne-makes it more effective)- may add tomatoes juice

-remove yellow peel of a grapefruit with potatoes peeler– cut thinly + 2 large garlic bulb- into 1 ½ qt. Water- cook till very bitter (about 20 minutes)- drink 1 cup every 20 minutes- may use along with enemas (by the time qt. Is done so is infection)

-combine a handful of peach leaves and half of handful of yarrow- mix with 2 grapefruits, 3 lemons, one large garlic bulb- cut out peelings cook till very bitter-drink ½ cup 3x daily

Supplement-Vitamin B complex, especially B6, B12, folic acid, and pantothenic acid. Vitamin E: 400-800 units

INDIGESTION

Do not eat too heavily of legumes, especially lentils, peanuts, and soybeans. They contain a substance which slows down certain digestive enzymes.

One cause is eating salads and other light food at the beginning of the meal, and waiting till partway through the meal to eat the protein foods. But protein foods need lots of hcl

Herbs- balm, bitter orange, celandine, hops, fennel, and yarrow.

Use "bitters"—aloe, angelica, bayberry root bark, and sparingly of Senna.

-1 tsp. Psyllium powder seeds + 3 tbs. Bentonite clay in apple juice- 3x daily

Diet-- Ginger ,Papain, papaya pineapple

Take lemon juice, diluted with water (or totally undiluted) at the beginning of each meal.

Comfrey fomentation- blend fresh comfrey and hot water in the blender- soak a handful in the solution. Wring out, fold once and place over the lower abdomen for 30 minutes. Use a hot fomentation over the top to keep it warm

Take colon cleanse

3 parts olive oil and 1part charcoal

Study show-cooked food and found that, when it was eaten, the white blood cells increased rapidly in the small intestine. Eating raw foods protects the immune system.

-1 heaping tbs. Of charcoal in a glass of water 3x daily -aloe Vera -take acidophilus or probiotics -chlorophyll heal	
INFECTION	
See immune section for rocket fuel **All infections:**-drink diluted grape juice through-out the day -grapefruit seed extract-2x daily -goldenseal caps- take 2 every 2 hours- till resolved Helpful herbs include Echinacea and goldenseal, Garlic is another powerful helper. **Take goldenseal and myrrh every** hour during fever **Antiseptic:** -1 clove of garlic blended in 1 cups of boiling water **Candida yeast:**- 2 tbsp. Acidophilus, 1 cup yo-gurt or acidophilus alone -garlic, goldenseal, paud'arco, psyllium, bee pol-len, passion flower, burdock, Echinacea, lobelia, ginger, gingko. Oregano grape -vitamin-a, e, b6, biotin **Fungal**- herbs -cranberry juice -aloe Vera juice 2 oz. 4 times daily-probiotics, caned, green apple, lime **Staph:**-vitamin-c, e, beta-carotene,, zinc-raw garlic, honeysuckle, bear lichen **Nail fungus** -Soak the feet for half an hour in a warm 1:5,000 solution of potassium permanganate. -*Pare and scrape the infected area*, and try to re-move as much of the loose material beneath the nails. Apply vinegar with a Q-tip twice a day. It may require months to eliminate. Fungus of the nails is the slowest to conquer.	**Sores** cabbage leaves poultice, Charcoal poultice- change poultice every 6-8 hours add flaxseed meal or boil 1 tbs. Flaxseed in 1 pt. Boiling water- then add charcoal -apply = part clay goldenseal+ honey/ aloe gel to consistency **Viral:** goldenseal, oranges, garlic, Echinacea, red raspberry-*chaparral **Systemic infection of** unknown cause:-treat as parasite (see herbs for worms, virus, bacteria, parasites)-give rocket fuel-charcoal hot bath for 1 hour- followed by 10 minutes cold tub or cold pour or cold hose -take charcoal water **Formula disinfectant spray:** 1 of each- grapefruit, lemon, lime, orange,+1tsp. Each- lemon oil, lime oil, eucalyptus oil+ 3 cups distilled water- blend and strain- peel all fruits except lemon (use for-fruit/ veg wash, wound care, sore throat, breath freshener,) *Supplement*- Zinc (50-100 mg daily Vitamins C, A, and B6
INFLAMMATION	
Inflammation that threatens gangrene: crushed marshmallow root as hot as possible add slip-pery elm to poultice(renew before it dries) **Herbs**- cayenne (externally) ,ginger	**Topical:**-4 cabbage leaves- place on top of each other and place on painful area -/ clay poultice -cover with paper towel and wrap with saran wrap leave overnight

MSM- for bones, joints, muscles **Teas**= hyssop, chickweed, vervain, mint, sage, bilberry, bromelain, Echinacea, devil's claw, feverfew, licorice root, onion ,goldenseal, paud'arco, red clover, ginger, *blue vervain	-charcoal poultice-clay pack-compress of fenugreek / chamomile -plantain leaf and keep plastic over it -witch hazel compress **Bromelin,** taken on an empty stomach and with a small amount of magnesium and L-cysteine

INSOMNIA

Check for calcium, potassium deficiency-check for parasites- causes multiple awakening during sleep especially between the hours of 2-3 am- check- b6 deficiency **Nervous and can't sleep:** compresses of wormwood/, balm/, chamomile, /lavender on the head **Nightmares:** -valerian root- simmers 1 tsps. In 1/2 cup water x 15 minutes let- cool- strain add water to 1/2 cups- drink before- bedtime -do not eat four hours before bed **Sleep apnea:** -sleep on sides -change life style **Formula:** -hops 2tbs -valerian 2 tbsp.-catnip 3tbs add to 1 qt. Water **Herbs-** hops, sage, or catnip tea **Tired, worn, nervous-**1st do hot foot bath with cold to head for 10 minutes then 60 degree wet sheet wrap and cover with blanket	**Hydrotherapy: do not -use hot and cold** (it is stimulating) apply a thick, warm (not hot) fomentation to spine for twenty minutes. Produce normal fatigue by daily exercise. A neutral bath at 44° to 97° will aid in reducing congestion of the brain and spinal cord, a very frequent accompaniment of insomnia *-fomentation to spine*(apply very warm not hot for 20-30minutes) the fomentation can also be applied to the spine, liver and stomach *-nervous exhaustion-* see wet sheet pack- cold water around neck -neutral bath for 1/2 hour before bed-hot abdominal pack at night Sleeplessness- 1 oz. Each- valerian, angelica, chamomile, sage- 1-2 tsp. In 1 cup boil h20-cool -1-2 cup sipping at night

INTESTINAL

Herbal-a=acute; sa=subacute; c=chronic; d=degenerative A-(colitis) goldenseal, garlic, slippery elm, marshmallow, capsicum, comfrey, valerian, lobelia Sa- (gas, constipation) alfalfa, goldenseal, cascara sagrada C-(bowel pockets) alfalfa, psyllium seed, cascara sagrada A-(degenerative stage) chaparral, Echinacea, goldenseal, yucca, comfrey, red clover, blue violet **Cramps:** catnip, flaxseed, tormentil, passion flower, rue, German chamomile	**Intestinal fermentation:** bilberry, alfalfa, angelica, a\anise, thyme, eucalyptus **Colic and stoppage of bowel:** lobelia + cayenne- 1 tsp, myrrh gum + valerian root 1tsp, make a stronginfusion of raspberry leaves -- then add the other herbs--mix , let stand tightly 1/2 hour and strain---inject 1/3 in rectum repeat the remainder in 4 hours **Bulky, pale, foul feces:** =malabsorption **Intestinal gas:** peppermint, cumin, tarragon, black poplar, fennel, caraway, garlic

IRRITABLE BOWEL SYNDROME

Cause-allergy, **Lactose-**intolerance-70%,Do not chew gum or smoke -avoid stress

Symptoms: change in bowel habits, abdominal pain, gas, nausea, lack of appetite, bad breath, heartburn, bloating, backache, weakness, faintness, palpitations may be present-20% has rectal bleeding-may have the following -constipation-pain, alternating constipation and diarrhea

Diarrhea usually occurs immediately upon arising, and after breakfast *"pencil like stool"*

Diet-Add crushed psyllium seed to your diet fat free, sugar free, eat at regular hours, don't drink fluids with meals; add bran daily to diet high fiber diet

TO PREVENT DIARRHEA- CAROB: mix 1-3 tablespoons carob powder in enough water to make a paste or put in your oatmeal at breakfast. Take 3 times a day at meals. Treat with charcoal: mix 1-3 tablespoons

Enema

FOR ABDOMINAL PAIN: heating pad, hot water bottle, and fomentations applied to the abdomen.

Bowel detox: 2 parts charcoal, 3 parts bentonite clay, 7 parts psyllium seed powder, 2 part marshmallow root powder, 1 part fennel powder stir 1 tbs. Into 1 glass of water or juice. Drink immediately. Do this 2-3x daily ½ hour before meals

HERBAL REMEDIES: chamomile, rosemary, balm, bayberry, gentian, skullcap, ginger, goldenseal, lobelia, marshmallow, pau d' Arco, rose hips, and valerian , acidophilus

Grape seed extract over four to six weeks. Grapefruit seed extract is also a good anti-fungal supplement. Put 4-8 drops of the grapefruit seed extract in each glass of water taken in. *Peppermint oil* (1 drop in ½ cup water)

JAUNDICE	
Neonatal- breast-fed more frequently, the bowel movements will carry bilirubin out of the body faster. Feed every 2 hours, in order to reduce bilirubin levels. *-activated charcoal-* stir 2-3 tsp. In a little water and give -begin at 4 hours of age-give every 4 hours for 120 hours-for premature infants- give x 168 hours give until bilirubin level drops to normal-may mix charcoal with breast milk-feed infant every 2 hours- carries bilirubin out through bowels-expose in sunlight through window (protect eyes) *-golden seal* –few drops in mouth until jaundice leaves	**Adult-**hot abdominal packs- fomentation for 15 min. Every 2-3 hours-sweating hot bath - for 15 minutes (steam bath, full bath)-wet sheet pack-followed by wet sheet rub *Itching*—neutral salt bath *Take-*a-drink copious amount of water. *Go on a liver flush* (apple juice alone for 3 days, followed by drinking a cup of olive oil and a cup of lemon juice)*herb:* - take 1 cups of goldenseal or Echinacea 1 hour before meals 3x daily-burdock root, agrimony, celandine, red clover, licorice, dandelion, chionathus, Swedish bitters-1 tbs. 3x daily and place compress of Swedish bitters over the liver *Extracted from the milk thistle,* helps repair damage to the liver*supplement:-*vitamin -c to bowel tolerance-vitamin-a, e, selenium, silymarin *Ginger syrup* (1 oz.) And 1 oz. Each of fluid extracts-of butternut and boneset- give 1tsp. 3-4x daily *Take -hot-high herb enema-*use white oak bark, bayberry bark
JOINTS	
A=acute; sa=subacute; c=chronic; d=degenerative A-(gout, bursitis, arthritis) alfalfa, burdock, comfrey Sa- (rheumatism) alfalfa, chaparral, oat straw C-(rheumatoid arthritis) capsicum, chaparral, black cohosh D-(osteoarthritis) chaparral, black cohosh, oat straw	

KIDNEY

Inflammation-Herbal-do not use parsley if with kidney inflammation a=acute; sa=subacute; c=chronic; d=degenerative

A-(acute nephritis) goldenseal, juniper berries, parsley, chaparral

Sa-(kidney stones) juniper berries, oat straw, valerian, ginger root

C-(chronic nephritis) goldenseal, chaparral, juniper berries

-Take a high enema and a daily hot half-hour tub bath. Give 2-3 cups of pleurisy tea or sage tea while in the tub. Finish with a short cold shower or cold towel rub. Do not allow them to get chill. Wrap him up well, put him in bed, and give him more pleurisy tea or sage tea to encourage perspiration. Fomentations over the lower back and the entire length of the spine will help alleviate pain.

Kidney formula

-4 oz. Beet juice 3x daily drink nothing butwater during the beets treatment- will usually response in 24 hours

-water fast -flax seed tea 2 tbs. In 1 glass of water boil x 5 minutes- cool and dilute take 1/2 glass of water every 2 hours for 2 days- coffee enema (see cleanse)-

-1/2 cups lemon juice blended with 1/2 olive oil (lay on right side for 30 minutes)--to avoid vomit suck on lemon take 1 hour after enema and take herbal laxative

-Suggested use is 2 or 3 capsules between meals, or a cup of tea morning and evening taken with a cup of parsley tea Ingredients: Juniper Berries-Parsley Root-Marshmallow Root-Golden Seal Root-UvaUrsi Leaf-Lobelia Herb-Ginger Root

Kidney disease, failure

In one study, one way to help the kidneys get rid of their wastes is by deep pool therapy. After 30 minutes with the kidney failure patient standing in a pool of water up to the shoulders, there was a diuresis of water, sodium, and potassium. The pool bath is much preferable to a tub bath in this regard

Kidney Infection -cranberry juice and apple juice

-hot trunk pack-followed by friction -fomentation to loins for 30 minutes every 3-4hours heating compress over lower back in the interval between-avoid cold full bath, cold douche

Supplement- vitamins C, A, and B complex in the diet. Potassium deficiencies can encourage kidney problems

-herbs include garlic, Echinacea, burdock, red clover, and goldenseal. Watermelon-seed tea. Buchu tea and marshmallow tea- huckleberry leaf-juniper -corn silk 3caps daily

-goldenseal 1/2 tsp 2x daily-juniper oil 10 drops 2x daily in 1 cups of yarrow tea

-dandelion 6 cap daily -alfalfa 5 cap 2x daily-peach leaf 1/2 ld. Of leaves to 1 quart water take 3 cups daily -

-drink lots of fluids -take enema 3x daily

Supplement: -vitamin -c, d, b- complex -potassium glutamate- potassium deficiency can encourage kidney problem

Kidney stones

Pain- full hot blanket pack=hot full bath, drink hot water- cool compress to head, neck and heart put hot moist blanket over a dry blanket-wrap around patient-put hot water bottle between legs, foot along the trunk tuck dry blanket to keep heat in- change compress every 10 minutes - treat x 30 min

Supplement-choline

-pain when passing stone: - 8 qt. Water- wrap a palm size ginger in a cloth, tied with a string -boil x 2-3 minutes.-reduce heat till boil stops-remove -squeeze and replace in pot -place on lower back on affected kidney-put plastic then cloth over area -repeat x 5-10 minutes x 30-45 minutes

-vomiting: - ice to throat

-urinary suppression: -hot blanket pack- followed by dry sweating pack

-kidney insufficiency- see heating compress to trunk

-*watermelon fast*

-*beets*- wash + slice 6-8 beets (medium) cook in 1 quart water ---refrigerate and take 3 glass daily or 4 oz. Beet juice 3x daily drink nothing but water during the beets treatment- will usually response in 24 hours

-*flax seed tea* 2 tbs. In 1 glass of water boil x 5 minutes- cool and dilute-take 1/2 glass of water every 2 hours for 2 days- coffee enema (see cleanse)-

-*1/2 cups lemon* juice blended with 1/2 olive oil (lay on right side for 30 minutes)-to avoid vomit suck on lemon take 1 hour after enema and take herbal laxative

-*Echinacea and goldenseal*

Kidney water retention: dandelion, corn silk, chickweed, horsetail, cleaver

Fever: carrot- beet juice

-*beet juice help remove stones* -vitamin-a prevents formation

-6-8 medium sized beets cook 6-8 medium beets, sliced cooked till tender in 1 qt. Water-strain- drink three glasses of this daily

-*To dissolve kidney stones*, drink hot water and lemon juice., *hydrangea and gravel root*

Kidney hydrotherapy:

-Congestion- hot packs with ice bags, b. Insufficiency and congested- full hot blanket

-Kidney stone- kidney stone pack=heating pad on top of sheet-hot fomentation on pad-plastic over -plug a radio in same outlet on high volume - static= water- danger-keep head cool

Dialysis-deep pool therapy .after 30 minutes with the kidney failure patient standing in a pool of water up to the shoulders, there was a diuresis of water, sodium, and potassium.

LARYNGITIS

Hydrotherapy- heating compress to throat-ice bag to the throat with general cold douche

*Take-*1 glass water + 1/2 tsp. Anise seed- boil x 15 minutes- strain+1/4 cup honey +4 tbs. Apple cider vinegar +1/2 tsp cayenne +1/2 tsp ginger powder use one tbs. As needed will restore voice

-mix 1 ld. Bran with ½ cup fructose and add 2 qt. Of boiling water-drink 1 cup throughout the day

-slippery elm+ honey and lemon

Singer's plant" is hedge mustard

-hedge mustard extract= singers plant -ginger, horehound, mullein the –eyebright

-2 tbs. Flaxseed + 1tbs horehound boil 1 pt. Water x 10 minutes- squeeze one lemon In the tea + pinch of ginger take 1 tbs. Every 1/2 hour

-Echinacea, plantain, knotgrass, primrose, white oak bark tea, marshmallow

-drink and gargle wild cherry bark tea / -gargle goldenseal

LEAKY GUT SYNDROME

Diet-:-cook grains in thermos jar (slow cooking is healing and is loaded with

Necessary nutrients)-in these juice (carrot, parsley, cabbage, -carrot, endive, ginger, -ginger, parsley, garlic, celery) drink almond milk-raw and steamed vegetables

A day or two of fasting per week

-one teaspoon slippery elm in water half an hour before each meal

Flavonoids before eating, (found in catechins, milk thistle, and dandelion root

Supplement-take acidophilus, papain and bromelain, beta-carotene, vitamin-b complex, vitamin-c, antioxidants, calcium, magnesium, flax oil, wheat germ oil, seaweed-acetyl glucosamine: 500 mg. 1 capsule, 2x a day.

Herbs-aloe Vera juice, grape seed extract, pau d'arco, cat's claw, licorice, slippery elm, comfrey, goldenseal

Slippery elm powder: 1 t. In ½ cup water. Stir well and take ½ hour before each meal. Following the

Glutathione (GSH) and n-acetyl cysteine (do not take these if you are taking artemisia or any other parasite medicine.) Use two pills of nag(n-acetyl glucosamine)three times a day for one year

Essential fatty acids (walnuts and flaxseed)

Whole grain at least once daily for the first six weeks after the discovery of a leaky gut

If a hidden infection is a probability-use goldenseal, Echinacea, artemisia, and garlic as anti-germ agents.

Candida **cleanse** 30-day *grapefruit seed extract* "cure" for *candida.* 15 drops of GSE three times a day.

LEUKEMIA

Symptoms:-weakness, weightloss, easy fatigue, remarkable whiteness of the skin, difficulty in-breathing, spells of fever, , slow healing cuts, palpitation, rapid heart, excessive seating, easy bruising, soreness or ulceration of the throat or gums, swollenlymph nodes, bone and joint pain, enlarge spleen or liver, tendency to hemorrhage or nosebleeds -effect both children and adults

Formula tea:-gentian 2 parts ,Irish moss -1 part, goldenseal 1/2 part, bayberry-2 part-fenugreek seed 2 part ,chickweed -1 part, comfrey - 2 part ,bugleweed -1 part

-yellow dock 1/2 part, prickly ash -1 part -St. John's wort 1 part (berries)-blue vervain 1 part, mandrake -1/3 part, evening primrose1 part, Echinacea -3 part

Cause: =cancer of the of one of the organs where the white blood cells are made (bone marrow, lymph system, or spleen)-blood forming organs are producing immature white blood cells or leucocytes

-these immature wbc's are too much and thus cause red blood cells amount to decrease-HIV, toxic exposure (radiation, radon, benzene etc.) -down syndrome-commercial hair dyes -poor living habits

Diet-beet juice -3 oz.

2x/d -alfalfa- 16capsuls daily-diet 85 %raw vegetables -. Km 3 oz. 2x daily

-*vegetable juice:* for 1-2 days-- organically grown-after first 2 days drink your juices- carrot drink 4 oz. Daily-broccoli 1part -Brussels sprouts juice 1 part-greens juice 1 part

-celery juice 1 part, mix above juices and drink 4 oz. 4 x daily

-*blend one cup of prunes* and add 1 gallon of grape juice let sit x 24 hours, refrigerate-- drink 2 oz. 2x daily, drink 2 oz. Beet juice 2x daily

Hydrotherapy- neutral baths daily x 2 weeks

Enema (garlic):3x daily -12 oz. Garlic per enemagarlic and onions --has anti platelet, blend 10 garlics bulbs in a little water and freeze let it thaw and eat 1 tsp3x daily-drink 2 cups onion tea daily

No enema cleanse (under 15 years old use 1 tsp)catnip enema 1x daily

Children: supplement: vitamin- e 400 iu. 2x daily, vitamin-A 25,000 iu. 2x daily (for 3 weeks), vitamin- B12 1000mg daily, vitamin-C 10,000mg 3x daily

-milk thistle 1/2 part(mix all together- take 8 capsules daily)

Daily herbs:astralagus 4cap 3x daily, shiitake 4 cap 3x daily, reishi 4 cap 3x daily black strap molasses 1 tbsp. 3x daily iron drink --see anemia

Green drink: -6 oz. Daily-a 25,000iu

Iron drink formula:-take 4 oz. 4x daily of the following mixture -black strap molasses, figs, apricots, raisins + prunes in large bottle of grape juice-let stand x 24hours, then refrigerate-eat the fruit when juice is finished

Mushroom is recommended for this disease -mix 1/4 tsp ginger powder, 1/4 tsp cayenne pepper + 1 cup of black mushroom- eat 1 tbsp. 3x daily

Supplement:-vitamin-e 2400 iu. Daily (rats lacking vitamin-e develops too many wbc's

-vitamin- b12- 2000mg daily -vitamin- b complex- 300mg daily -wheat germ- 1tsp 2x daily

-vitamin-d - 1000mg daily -vitamin-c - 10,000 mg daily -for children 2,000mg daily

-multi vitamin. Calcium and mg. -vitamin -a 25,000iu 2x daily (for 3 weeks)-laetrile, germanium, selenium,

-quercetin, genistein**found in citrus pulp destroys leukemia cells

-bioflavonoids = sources include (peppers, buckwheat, black currant, white

Material just beneath of citrus fruits, citrus pulp, cherries, apricots,

Blackberries, plums, prunes, rose hips)

LICE-See "BITE " section	
LIVER	

Symptom-white or pale stools signify disease of the liver, liver cirrhosis-check copper deficiency

Herbs-a=acute; sa=subacute; c=chronic; d=degenerative

A-(acute hepatitis) chaparral, lobelia, dandelion, yarrow, mandrake, comfrey root

Enema-hot colonic- at 105 followed by small cold enema 2x daily- fomentation over liver and stomach every 2 hours (during the interval -heating compress - change every 30 min.)

-*enema 3x daily-coffee 3tbs* ground coffee to 1 quart water 2x weekly

Sa-(sluggish, congested) mandrake, cayenne, goldenseal, chaparral

C-(chronic hepatitis) dandelion root, chaparral, burdock, Echinacea

D-(cirrhosis) burdock, cascara sagrada, goldenseal, mandrake

-chlorophyll- purifies liver

-milk thistle- liver detox-wheat grass- regenerates the liver

SEE CASTOR OIL PACK (cleanse section)

Hydrotherapy-(HOT LIVER PACK over liver area) -blend 2 grapefruits -with 1 1/2 cups of Epson salt.-pour mixture on large cotton towel -wrap towel tight to prevent mixture from escaping -rub the area over the liver with olive oil -then place the pack-put a hot bottle over the pack x 30 minutes -leave pack on overnight(steam bath 2 or more times weekly)c. Hot Epson salt bath 3x daily

-*sluggish liver*-see fomentation -see wet sheet pack (cooling stage)

-*congestion*- see wet sheet pack (heating stage)

-*jaundice*- see wet sheet pack(neutral stage)

-*inflamed*- burdock leaf pack over liver

Diet-*beets and spinach*3-7 day detox program:

Lemon-4 medium mixed in 1 1/2 quarts of distilled water take in morning and at

Bedtime-3 oz. Beet juice 2x daily or 8 beet tab. 3x daily-drink 1 or 2 quarts carrot juice daily, drink 1 pint of green juice 2x daily

Potassium high foods- kelp, and dulse, rice, bananas, blackstrap molasses, wheat bran, almonds, seeds, brewer's yeast, prunes and raisins

heating trunk pack- for these conditions 20-25 minutes is the usual treatment time.

Overdose-liver failure activated charcoal use as much as possible both internally and externally. A charcoal and water mixture was applied to the back, abdomen and chest, and also introduced orally

-*hot herb enema 2x* daily- use white oak bark or bayberry bark tea

Formula-liver-and-gallbladder-Dosages:

Suggested dose: 1/3 Cup or one or two capsules or tablets, 15 to 20 minutes before a meal.

- 4oz. Ginger syrup + 1oz. Each of extract-butternut, and boneset--- give 1 tsp 3-4 x daily*

-barberry 2 tbs. Cramp bark 2 tbs., catnip 1 tbsp., liverwort 3 tbs., chamomile 1 tbsp. Gentian 3 tbsp. Red beet 2 tbsp., parsley 3 tbsp. (mix and use 2 tbs. In 6 oz. Of hot water – drink3x daily)

-mixed 1 to 1 ½ qt. Of soft distilled water take in the morning and before bedtime-8 bran tablets -3 times daily,

Liver lymphatic flow and liver activity. 1 clean whole lemon (pulp, rind, seeds, and all)

1 tablespoon of extra virgin olive oil _1 ½ cups of distilled water

4 rounded tablespoons of frozen orange juice concentrate, strain through a wire strainer to remove the pulp, and discarded. Divide in four equal portions of approximately ¼ cup each and a portion is consumed with each of the three daily meals and before bedtime

Liver spots-Swedish bitters compress to area

Jaundice:-goldenseal extract- few drops in mouth till jaundice disappear

-5-6 lemons in 1 1/2 quart of water for 3 days then cut back to 4 lemons in 1 1/2 quart of water x 10 days then cut back to 2 lemons

Itching of skin- boric acid water

Liver flush-apple juice fast x 3 days-then 1 cup olive oil and 1 cup lemon

LIVER CIRRHOSIS

Pain-fomentation; revulsive compress or revulsive douche, with hot leg bath or hot leg pack, followed by compress over liver, twice daily

Avoid cold full baths and very cold general or prolonged cold douche

Enlarged liver- cascara sagrada*

Silymarin- 200mg 3x daily -drink 1/4 cup aloe Vera each morning

Diet- **liver building juice:** 6 lemon + 1cup molasses, 2 tbsp. Beet powder,1/2 tsp cayenne,4 tbsp. Alfalfa, 12 oz. Water-mix together

Supplement:-choline, inositol, cobalt vitamin-k (140mg), vitamin-a, zinc (30mg)-lemon, coenzyme q10, lecithin -dandelion, ginger, turmeric, rosemary, celandine, silymarin

-Silymarin helps the liver.

Herbs include burdock, celandine, barberry, Echinacea, goldenseal, fennel, red clover, and thyme

sluggish liver:- safflower*

Bleeding-vit-k-140mcg

Liver flush -yellow root

LIVER FAILURE

SEE CASTOR OIL PACK

Liver lymphatic flow and liver activity. 1 clean whole lemon (pulp, rind, seeds, and all) +1 tablespoon of extra virgin olive oil 1 ½ cups of distilled water +4 rounded tablespoons of frozen orange juice concentrate

Blend- strain discard pulp the remaining liquid is divided in four equal portions of approximately ¼ cup each and a portion is consumed with each of the three daily meals and before bedtime. OR

-1 grated beet, 1 tablespoon extra-virgin olive oil, and the juice of 1 lemon (include the peel and seeds if you like). *Add castor oil packs (usually for one hour a day)*

4 oz. Beet juice 3x daily-will usually response in 24 hours and take a coffee enema(see cleanse) -1/2 cups lemon juice blended with 1/2 olive oil(lay on right side for 30 minutes)-to avoid vomit suck on lemon take 1 hour after enema and take herbal laxative

Take coffee enema- 1 hour after enema --take 1 glass lemon juice+1/2 glass olive oil lie on right side x 30 minutes. (suck on lemon to avoid vomit.

LOCKJAW

Grind peach leaves: apply to wound-2x daily

Turpentine: massage to jaw and put on wound, neck, jaw and spine

Wood ash: 2 cups to 1 gallon water and soak area

Tincture: (see epilepsy) 10 drops every 15 minutes if no tincture tobacco poultice over stomach

Lobelia tincture and cayenne 1 tsp every 15 minutes if no tincture: 1 tsp lobelia + 1 qt. Water boil with 1 tsp cayenne let stand x20 minutes take 1/4 cup every 1/2 hour

Rub antispasmodic tincture around clenched jaw

LUNGS

atelectasis-URGENT call 911-=collapse lung-sudden sever shortness of breath, chest pain,/ tightness

Respiratory protection: wild cherry bark, lobelia, skullcap, licorice, lungwort, Irish moss, elecampane, yerba mate, buckthorn, black root,

Pneumothorax- sudden severe shortness of breath, chest pain,/ tightness chest pain, sharp pain @ *1 side of chest at deep*

Pulmonary edema - cough, *shortness of breath,* productive cough (pink frothy sputum)

Pulmonary embolism cough, *blood sputum, chest pain sudden shortness of breath, pedal and leg edema,* fever, shortness of breath, coughing up mucus/ blood

Herb-lungs/bronchial-a=acute;

Sa=subacute; c=chronic; d=degenerative

A-(coughs, colds) mullein, horehound, slippery elm, wild cherry bark

Sa-(bronchitis) catnip, comfrey, goldenseal, mullein, yarrow, myrrh

C-(asthma) blue vervain, horehound, comfrey, coltsfoot, marshmallow, valerian

D-(Hodgkin's) cayenne, goldenseal, chaparral, Echinacea

Formula lung & bronchial-Suggested amount for an adult is a cup two or three times a day, or two or three capsules or tab. 2 – 3 times a day with a cup of comfrey tea. Opt. Adds three to six drops of tincture of lobelia to each cup of tea. Ingredients: comfrey leaves-mullein-chickweed-marshmallow root-lobelia

Formula: mullein- 1part, marshmallow-1part, comfrey- 1part, slippery elm- 1part, lobelia- 1/2 part, peppermint oil 1/2 tsp(mix make tea with 2tbs) take daily **or**

-1/2 tsp. Peppermint oil+ 1 tbs. Garlic + 1cup honey- mix and use ½ tsp. As needed

Supplement: vitamin b17 (nitrilosides)- used to treat lung infection, flaxseed oil

Stronger lungs: celandine, rosemary, angelica, buckthorn, speedwell wild plum and centaury, cramp bark*

sarsaparilla, yellow dock, burdock root, anise, *burnet

Shortness of breath:vervain*

Congestion of the lung -*onion & cornstarch-*, take a little oil in a skillet and add about a cup of onions. Take a little cornstarch (just enough to thicken it). As you are stir frying you want to keep adding some cornstarch to it to be. Make it real thick. Use a lot of paper towels OR chucks cut it in half when I do a poultice. Take the flax seed or charcoal poultice and put it under the cotton layer and mash it flat. Put the cotton side toward the body and the plastic side out to protect it. Take these onions and cover it over. Make it like a pocket so that it won't fall out. Then apply it to the chest

-hydrotherapy- fomentations for chest congestion, hot and cold chest bath steam bath 3x / week, fever bath 2x/ week-fomentations to back followed by cold compresses

Cold compress to chest and back with hot leg pack -clay bath if strong enough

Hemorrhage:-pulmonary ice pack to chest- remove and dry with warm dry flannel for 1-2 minutes every 15 minutes-hot leg pack -very hot sponging of upper 1/2 of the spine-place hands in ice water for 1-2 minutes-after hemorrhage ceases- graduated cold treatment to increase resistance to disease that caused bleeding

Diet- eat lots of kiwi

LUPUS

Symptoms: joints and blood vessels are affected producing arthritis-like symptoms, kidneys and lymph nodes become inflamed. In severe cases there is heart, brain, and central nervous system degeneration. The skin and kidneys can be affected

Juice:8 oz. Carrot juice, 4 oz. Celery juice, 4 oz. Beet juice, 1 cup alfalfa sprout1 tsp kelp (drink 16 0z. Fresh 1-2 x daily)-16 oz. Grape juice (with seed), 16 oz. Unsweetened juice and ½ cup sunflower seeds. Mix together.-1 tsp. Flax seeds, 1 tsp. (whole) in food or drink

Causes:=autoimmune disease- the body's own immune system , starts attacking the connective tissues -lupus means "wolf"- because of the roughness of the skin of the cheeks and nose of some victims -birth control pills, corticosteroid drugs, penicillin, allergenic cosmetics, UV rays- any of these can cause a flare up of lupus*parasite is associated with lupus do parasite cleanse*

allergies are also associated with lupus

Diet-: -drink 48 oz. Water daily -raw diet and juicing-drink plenty of water

-60-75% fresh foods -take potassium broth for 1 months - from thick potatoes peeling

-garlic -low fat diet, cabbage juice, olives, flaxseed and flaxseed oil (1-3teaspoons, 1-3 times daily), celery (3 stalks pureed once or twice a day), nightshade free for 3 months trial (tomatoes, potatoes, eggplant, peppers, pimento, paprika), and gluten grains omitted (wheat, rye, barley, oats). Pineapple suppresses inflammation; so do apples and hawthorn berry tea.

Avoid eating alfalfa sprouts, for they contain canavain which, in your body, replaces its arginine.

-Protein drink- mix 8 oz. Of soy milk, 1 tbs. Of sunflower seed, 1 tbs. Of alfalfa seeds-blend together- drink 2 times daily

Supplement: -kyolic garlic- 5 capsules 3x daily -vitamin-c 1000mg daily-vitamin -a 25,000 iu. 2x daily -sarsaparilla 8 cap. 2x daily-blackstrap molasses- 1 tbsp. 2x daily am + pm -kelp 10 capsule daily -flaxseed oil 1tbs daily-vitamin b5 (panthotenic acid) -PABA-take 1-2 glasses of aloe Vera juice daily-alfalfa tablets to increase fiber -vitamin-e

Herbs: formula:-2 oz. Paud'arco -1 oz. Chaparral -1 oz. Black walnut -1 oz. Red clover (mix 1 tsp per cup. Boil water- steep x 15 minutes) (let cool strain- drink 4-6cups daily without sweetener)

LYME-SEE "bite" SECTION (TICKS)	
LYMPH	

See "glands" section

Symptoms: -swelling of lymph nodes (commonly referred to as glands)-some locations (neck, throat, armpits, groins)

Causes: -lymph nodes filter the infections -infection in lymph by (measles, chicken pox, mononucleosis, TB, syphilis, leukemia, cancer) cat scratch disease

Apply- **poultice-apply to area teas of:**-comfrey/, plantain/, apple cider vinegar and witch hazel-use one or more-poultice; carrot/ castor oil packs/ lavender lotion or lavender water/ parsley tea

Pregnancy- they also apply 2 parts turmeric and 1 part salt to area

Diet--drink 2-3 qt. Water daily -5- 14 days fruit juice fast-high potassium diet (potatoes, onions, carrots, banana)

Herbs: -garlic enema 3x daily-take a cleanser 5x daily -goldenseal -2 cap 2x daily -Echinacea -10 cap daily-pau d'arco- 10 cap daily -garlic- blend 5 bulbs with a little water- take 1 tsp 5x daily -ocotillo, myrrh, red root, Echinacea, goldenseal

-in India- ginger has been used for centuries-take 2 oz. Daily (results within 30 days)-do not take during

- compress of strong decoction of rue tea

-compress -2 oz. Mullein, 1/2 oz. Lobelia powder, 1 tsp. Cayenne. Simmer in 2 qt. Apple cider vinegar, cover for 15 min., strain, and apply with wool

Supplement:-calcium- 1,500 mg daily -iron- see anemia formula -silicon -vit-c 20,000mg daily-red clover- drink like water -yellow dock- 5 caps 3x daily

Hydrotherapy-skin brushing excellent. Salt glow-steam bath daily 1x for 10 days or fever bath daily x 10 days then 3x weekly alternate with fever bath

Cleanse; drinking a combination of olive oil and lemon juice to further stimulate lymphatic flow and liver activity. It can be made by blending the following:1 clean whole lemon (pulp, rind, seeds, and all)

1 tablespoon of extra virgin olive oil+1 ½ cups of distilled water 4 rounded tablespoons of frozen orange juice concentrate 2-3 qt. Water daily-

Formula: 1part=1tbs.(mix the following take 6 capsules 2x daily)gentian 3 part ,yellow dock 1 part bayberry bark 1 part, prickly ash 1 part, golden seal1 part , St. John's wort 1 part, Irish moss 1 part ,blue vervain 1 part, comfrey 2 part, mandrake 1 part milk thistle 2 part , pau d'arco 3 part

-potassium glucanate-99mg 5x daily -iodine in liquid or capsules- 10 capsules of kelp daily-zinc lozenges -every 2 waking hours for 1 more week, then 50 iu. For 30 days

*chaparral+ better when combined with Echinacea

-fenugreek and garlic- detox the lymph-clover tea- drink all day like water

-goldenseal- 2 cap 2x daily- beta-carotene-200,000 iu. Daily x 2 weeks -then 100,000 iu.-echenesea- 10 cap daily -paud'arco- 10 cap daily -vitamin-b complex important

-garlic blend 5 cloves and take 1 tsp 5x daily -red root- long term lymphatic cleanse

-400-500 mg pure pineapple compound (from health food store) 3x daily on an empty stomach

MALNUTRITION	
Distended abdomen= liver swelling, nails yellow= nutritional deficiency	**Magnesium therapy**
MEMORY	
Unclear thinking- check for parasites **recent memory loss not Alzheimer's:** -check for b-1 deficiency-vitamin- b1, chromium/vanadium, selenium, betaine HCL **Swedish bitters-** put at base of scalp **delirium-** heating wet sheet pack -ice cap to head -prolonged sweating wet sheet pack	**Hysteria-** throw in cold pool while unsuspected **Supplements:**-ginkgo, gotu kola, ginseng, mullein oil -acetyl-l-carnitine -lecithin -l-tyrosine-boron 3mg daily -pycnogenol -60mg 3x daily -melatonin- 2-3 mg take 2-3 hours beforebedtime **Herbs:** blue cohosh, gotu kola, blessed thistle, valerian, anise
MENINGITIS *is CONTAGIOUS*	
<u>**Meningitis can progress quickly**</u> and become life threatening in 24 hours for adults and even quicker For children. Call a physician **symptoms:** varies - take to emergency room contagious-sore throat, fever, headache, stiff neck, and vomiting-may become critical within 6-24 hours of first onset of symptoms -sore throat, red or purple skin, rash, fever, chills, malaise, headache, vomiting, sensitivity to light, nausea, delirium, stiff neck, convulsions *-infants-vomiting,* fever, difficulty feeding, irritability, high-pitched cry, bulging fontanel (soft spot on head), changes in temperature, extreme sleepiness indicates dangerous changes in cerebrospinal fluid **Cerebral meningitis-** immerse back of head in warm Epson salt solution severaltimes daily to draw out inflammation **Headache:** fomentation to back of neck, ice compress to head and neck, hot and cold head compress **Muscular rigidity—**hot blanket pack; hot full bath; hot fomentation, followed by well-protected heating compress **Muscle spasm:** hot full bath at 102 degrees for 15- 30 minutes-prolongs neutral bath, heating spinal compress	**Spinal meningitis-** fomentation to spine, liver and abdomen-rest in bed , with a very dim light, at the most), well-ventilated room, no visitors, drink plenty of liquid-compresses of Swedish bitters to back of head **Massage** hastens recovery **Herbs-**a=acute; sa=subacute; c=chronic; d=degenerative D-(MS, meningitis) comfrey, chaparral, evening primrose, sarsaparilla, grape juice **Herb-** goldenseal, Echinacea, 6-8 garlic tablets daily, skullcap, gotu kola teas **Supplement:** niacinamide (100-500mg daily), vitamin-a (400iu for children and 5,000 iu. For adults),- b6(100mg), B12 (2,000mcg), B- complex ,-C(1/2 tsp. Every 1/2 hour during acute phase: reduce by 1/2 maintenance tillcomplete recovery) **Diet-** acute- don't eat, citrus juices, fresh pineapples helps reduce the infection Drink citrus juices, from lemons, oranges, and limes. **Fever-** catnip enema+ sip the tea **High herbal(catnip) enema -** must have a bowel movement 2-3x daily **Hydrotherapy-**careful cold mitten friction, 2-4 times daily

-alternate-hot and cold packs on neck and back of the head to stimulate circulation to the area, plus fomentation to liver and abdomen **Pain in back and legs**—fomentation to back; hot hip pack. Repeat every 4 hours or more often. Heating compress or ice bag during interval between.	Do not use cold full baths and other general cold procedures. *-ice cravat,* cool sponge baths , cooling compress to head, ice pack to spinehot hip packs, hot leg packs- with ice cap, fomentation to spine every 2 hours-cold mitten friction

MENSTRUAL DISORDERS

Note-Taking the birth control pill greatly upsets the entire hormonal system, and it does not recover, even after the pill is stopped for many months or years. - Problems with the pituitary, adrenals, or thyroid may produce amenorrhea, or abnormal bleeding cycles. Stress or the birth control pill can seriously affect the adrenals (which produce 20% of the total estrogen used by the body). **Excessive menstruation** amaranth and lady's mantle cycles. **Cramping** may be relieved by additional intake of calcium and niacin.-hot foot bath-peppermint tea *Due to ovarian disease* (beginning before flow)—hot hip and leg pack; hot blanket pack; fomentation over stomach; hot pelvic pack; revulsive sitz; hot colonic, followed by hot footbath if flow is checked; hot douche at 99⁰-102⁰ f.; very hot full bath (105⁰-110⁰ f.) For 5-8 minutes. *Due to uterine disease* (beginning with, and accompanying, flow)—hot hip pack with hot footbath, followed by cold compress to area above stomach and inner surfaces of thighs for 30-40 seconds. For treatment between periods, *Due to inflammatory* disease of appendages— hot enema, hot fomentations, hot pelvic pack, hot blanket pack	**Suppressed menstruation** life root, black cohosh, garlic and motherwort ephedra viridis -tonic sitz bath; cold pelvic pack; graduated baths, twice daily, for tonic purposes; short very cold douche to lower spine, over stomach, and to inner surfaces of thighs; pelvic massage daily, and especially when period is due. *Hydrotherapy-*take a daily hot sitz Bath. If available, add chamomile or juniper needles to the water. Or take two hot baths each day at the beginning of menstruation. This draws blood from the over-congested uterus to the skin. -a hot sitz bath (105°-115° f.) With a hot footbath (110°-117° f.) For 3-10 minutes is often helpful **Herbs-** blue cohosh, uvaursi, burdock, dong quai, goldenseal, chaparral, cohosh *-Drink catnip* tea each morning and evening during the period. *-chamomile* relieves menstrual spasms **Supplements-**Include B complex, especially B_{12} and B_6; along with vitamins C and E. Take brewer's yeast, kelp, and essential fatty acids. *-Iron is vital because* of the loss of blood each month. Vitamin C helps the body absorb iron-*Beware* of supplemental iron during pregnancy! Iron-rich sources include blackstrap molasses (best single source), apricots, and raisins. *Take vitamin A* as beta-carotene during the last 14 days of the cycle. *Vitamin B_{12}* helps restore normal menstrual

MENOPAUSE

Note- Hypothyroidism is common during menopause , Avoid mental and emotional stress and worry. Be happy with the blessings you have, and thank God for them.	**Herbs** include lady's mangle, motherwort, and St. John's wort. Nova Scotia dulse or Norwegian kelp.

Supplement-Vitamin E (up to 1,200 IU daily) is especially important at this time. Vitamin D, iron, and magnesium. Vitamin C, working with bioflavonoids, maintains capillary strength. B complex vitamins, especially pantothenic acid and PABA, relieve nervous irritability	**After menopause begins**, due to the lessened estrogen you will not have as much calcium in your body, it is important that you supplement with calcium.

MENTAL ILLNESS

Check deficiency (calcium, potassium - magnesium –delusions) *-many mental illness-* with too much lead and copper in the body **Supplement-**vitamin -b complex (especially b3,b6,b12 and folic acid) reduces excess estrogenfrom liver and prevents it from causing mental troubles -vitamin-e helps brain to get sufficient oxygen from lungs -lack of calcium- causes -vitamin-c 5000 daily, -glutamine 2 caps daily, - vitamin-b6 200mg 2x daily-gotu cola 3 cap 2x daily -lecithin 1 tbs. 3x daily -gingko 4 cap 3x daily tenseness -magnesium deficiency causes the person to be withdrawn, apathetic, uncooperative, belligerent- **Excessive compulsive behavior-** noni **Barley green** helps to cure mental problems **Cleanser:-**enema 3x weekly – cleanser -drink 2-3 qt. Of water daily	**Hydrotherapy-**the neutral sitz bath between 90° and 97° has a calming effect. It may be used in persons who are irritable or nervous for any reason, in itching, in mental illness, etc. **Herbs**: see nerves, gingko bilboa, hops, skullcap, valerian, wood betony, noni -formula#1-use = parts -valerian -hops -skullcap -catnip(mix - use 1 tbsp. In 6 oz. Water drink 3 cups daily)- -formula **#2** -alfalfa -1part, -black cohosh -1 part, -chickweed -1 part, -Echinacea -2 part, -kelp -2 part, -sarsaparilla -2 part, -red clover -2 part(mix- use 3 tbsp. To8 oz. Water +tea take 1 cup daily)

MONONUCLEOSIS IS *very contagious*

Symptom:-depression, fatigue, fever, generalized aching, sore throat, swollen glands, headache, jaundice, with possible red rash with raised bumps -similar to flu but symptoms last for 2-4 weeks-general fatigue for 3 weeks to years -severe dangerous symptoms - fever more than 102 f., **Cause:-**contagious disease primarily affecting the spleen and lymph -contracted bykissing, sex, sharing food or utensils. Do not strain at the stool, for this could injure a temporarily enlarged spleen.	**Stay in bed until the worst part is over. You need lots of rest** *Take-* take trace minerals dandelion tea, Echinacea *Diet-:* -fast (fruit and vegetable juicing for 2-3 days -eat a nourishing diet-vegetable soups, potatoes peeling broth, brown rice-severe sore throat- softdiet -take distilled water only Do not eat processed, or junk, food. Do not eat meat, sugar, fried foods, or drink soft drinks *Hydrotherapy-* give 30 minutes of *fever therapy* for 3 days (maintain body

Be alert to signs that a more serious splenic infection may be about to begin: a fever over 102° F, severe pain in the _middle of your left_ Side that last 5 minutes or more, breathing and swallowing becomes difficult, If this happens, contact your physician	Temperature at 102-103 f.) Use with hot foot baths- this produce dramatic results especially in advance cases

MOUTH / TEETH/ GUMS

Herbs- a=acute; sa=subacute; c=chronic; d=degenerative

A-(cold sores) comfrey, myrrh, sage, goldenseal

Sa-(cracked, chapped lips, tongue coating) comfrey, wintergreen, white oak bark, black walnut

C-(halitosis) alfalfa, goldenseal, parsley, myrrh

D-(degenerative stage) chaparral, Echinacea, comfrey. Alfalfa

A-(bleeding/ gingivitis) myrrh, goldenseal, comfrey root

Sa-(loose) myrrh, ipecac root, pomegranate

C-(caries) arbor vitae, myrrh

D-(pyorrhea) bayberry root and bark, goldenseal, rhatany root

Check for deficiency- calcium, phosphorus , molybdenum deficiency, see scurvy- vitamin-c deficiency- swelling and bleeding gums, see mouth cancer-feelings something stuck in tongue, patches, persistent sores, see diphtheria- greyish membrane forms in mouth and throat

Abscess: a-vitamin-c 1000mg every 1 hour for 4 days-pack chlorophyll around the teeth

-formula: -charcoal -2 part-goldenseal -1 part -myrrh -1 part -cayenne -1/2 part

-peppermint oil -2 drops -clove tincture -2 drops (make poultice and hold on abscess area)take: garlic 10 pearls 3x daily

Bad breath-check gum/ bowel disease

Need cleanse

Take charcoal by mouth. Let them dissolve slowly in the mouth.

Use myrrh, rosemary, or peppermint to brush your teeth and rinse your mouth.

Bruxism (teeth grinding)- check parasite

Saliva problems- The chewing gum habit is not good.

-_dry mouth,_ take a little lemon juice or honey before the meal

-_too much saliva,_ drink a tea of one of the following: white oak bark, goldenseal root, or bayberry.

-_See mucus section_ (check for-_Sjogren's Syndrome_)

Sore mouth: -1 oz. Bayberry bark, 1/2 oz. Blue cohosh +witch hazel and goldenseal- steep x 30 minutes-promotes healing: St. John's wort tea-

Sore gums-wash area bistort root tea* -toothbrush-twigs of flowering dogwood*

Stained teeth-brush with charcoal, polish teeth with baking soda, electric toothbrush

-remove tartar- mix equal part sea salt, baking soda and clean the teeth

Swelling and bleeding gum-see scurvy

-formula extracts of: calendula, olive leaf, Echinacea, ginseng, aloe, papaya, strawberry, guar gum, folic acid, zinc picolate, + oils of the following-spearmint, clove, eucalyptus, myrrh

-bleeding **sprinkle alum to area***-rinse mouth out with bistort root tea- it will give strength to gums

Tartar: mix = part cream of tartar, baking soda, sea salt, and clean teeth

Teeth grinding (bruxism)-check for parasites

-cause- stress, anxiety, anger, hypoglycemia, idle chewing on something- can lead to TMJ

-vitamin-C, zinc, calcium, pantothenic acid,-take at bedtime: valerian, skullcap, hops chamomile, teeth clenching- vitamin-B (panthotenic acid)

Cracks on corner of mouth /geographic tongue and cracks in corner nose, top side of tongue are irregular, appear smooth- not painful, sense of taste not effected-_causes_ :celiac disease- vitamin -B2 deficiency---means you are not absorbing B3, B6, b5, B12, folic acid, zinc -take B2 (500mg), B3 (200mg), B5 (2000mg), B12 (1000mg),folic acid (5mg), zinc(30mg)

Dry mouth- -vitamin-a deficiency could be a problem take - beta- carotene (5000mg)-lemon juice or honey before meals: rinse mouth with golden seal, Echinacea tincture to juice take co-enzyme Q-10 (10-30 mg daily), jaborandi, B-complex vitamins, aloe Vera- put on gums - do not eat for 1 hour after, cayenne, vitamin-c 2000mg daily-check for sjogren's syndrome

-drink at least 2 glasses of warm water 15-30 minutes before each meal

-take a little lemon juice and honey before meals

-vitamin -a deficiency may be a cause - take beta-carotene (5000iu)

Dry socket- analgesic herbs to area

Gingivitis -brush teeth with peroxide and / baking soda-rinse mouth with warm chamomile tea after each brushing of teeth. Powdered charcoal for several months brush with it- gingivitis (inflamed) chamomile, Echinacea, sage-grapefruit seed extract- powerful wheat grass- chew

Gum/ mouth problem: myrrh, propolis, Echinacea, goldenseal, bayberry

Bloodroot, gargle vinegar water

Infection-_mouthwashes:_ salt water -bistort -chamomile -got kola- good for gum healing- rinse and do not swallow rinse of hot peach pit tea-t-tree oil, witch hazel and calendula extract also

-mix aloe Vera and myrrh and apply it to the gums-lobelia extract

-drink 3 tsp chlorophyll liquid, and apply directly to gum

-brush teeth with- black polar powder mixed with charcoal

-t-tree oil 4-5 drops or grapefruit seed extract in a water pick daily

Tooth extraction; cayenne on gauze to area stops bleeding

Tooth sensitive. Calcium hydroxyapatite- restores teeth enamel and

Makes teeth less sensitive-mix= 1/4 tsp clove powder with few drops water put on sensitive tooth after each mea-mix =liquid extract= part fennel, white oak bark, horsetail- put few 7drops on

Sensitive tooth (put use as mouth rinse)

Toothache-rinse mouth with lukewarm water vigorously floss gently, salt water wash oil of cloves- crush garlic or grated horseradish on the tooth

-cayenne or pinch of cayenne and ginger in a little water- soak cotton ball and place in area- put charcoal tap on area- ginger ground in mouth then spit out

-grated horseradish- chew catnip herbs- 1-2 cups mullein tea

-chaparral-switch tea or chew and spit herb

-sesame- 1part to 2 part water boil till 1/2 the liquid is gone- apply to area

-myrrh-helps control mouth infection

-make paste with clove oil and zinc oxide- will protect cavity from food

-put heat at face area where toothache is located, chew willow bark

-ice rub to area, *hops tea- hold this herb in the mouth*blue false indigo

-apply-mash up plantain root

- soak a brown paper bag with vinegar and put outside cheek at side of pain

-sesame- boil 1 part to 2 parts water- boil till half the liquid is gone- apply to tooth, sprinkle a little cayenne and vinegar in water and switch around in the mouth -hold double strength sage tea in the mouth and swallow-1-2 cups of mullein tea or chew catnip herb

- hold 2 tbs. Of Swedish bitters with a little water in the mouth

-cayenne and garlic- apply pinesap to area

-inflammation: white oak bark

-.other helps: -rub-viamint-e oil (400iu) and or vitamin-a oil(500iu) on gum

-folic acid solution as a mouth wash

- pain: massage gums with diluted clove oil, diluted, eucalyptus oil , or lobelia

Lip balm -1 cup almond oil + in a double boiler-stir continuously-add 1 tbsp. Beeswax -add 1 tsp each of the following vanilla extract, honey vitamin-e oil, aloe Vera gel -while hot stir as you pour into wide mouth jar-close tightly

Leukoplakia-white, painless patches to tongue, rinse with aloe juice or a mixture of vinegar2tbs. And water rinse + a pinch of cayenne

-switch and swallow teas of -white oak bark/ myrrh/ goldenseal/ red raspberry

-wipe patches with cloth dipped in solution of borax mixed with water and honey

Loss of sense of taste- vitamin supplements, copper supplement

Oral thrush:paud'arco, goldenseal, bloodroot, yellow root, barberry, oregano grape, apply black walnut extract, t-tree to area, wild oregano oil to area, pepper tree, licaria puchuri-major

-use acidophilus and leave in mouth (use powder/ liquid)

Pyorrhea(gum disease)-goldenseal powder and myrrh powder - poultice apply to gum ,take- co enzyme q10, quercetin, bromelain, lysine-take supplements- calcium(2000mg), copper (4mg),vitamin-D (1000mg), C(2000mg), folic acid (5mg), niacin (2000mg), bioflavonoids (100mg)-take coenzyme Q10 (60mg, 2x daily) for almost immediate relief

-inflammation- quercetin and bromelein plus lysine, wheat grass- chew

Tooth decay-check vitamin-d deficiency (get from sun) -bay leaf - licorice wild, bergamot -blood root helps reduce plaque on teeth

-do not eat rhubarb and poke and spinach- high in oxalic acid- inhibits calcium-formation -goldenseal as a mouthwash

Ulcers in mouth: comfrey and burdock root and add 1 tsp boiling water steep and use

-pau d'arco 1 tbs.+ goldenseal 1 tbs. + burdock 1 tbs. Mix together and take 1 tsp.4x daily

-drink 3 cups of red raspberry tea daily- mix 3 tsp. Of herb per cup of water

-vitamin e and a gel gives relief – apply to area

-charcoal tablets may be used as throat lozenges, or as mouth lozenges in the case of mouth ulcers.

-garlic ear oil 1 drop 2x daily-proven to treat fungus better than drugs (1 cup chopped garlic. Cover with 2 cups cold pressed olive oil. Let sit for 7 days, shake daily. Strain oil into dark glass bottle with a top .store in fridge

Weak teeth -Irish moss**

Formula-barberry root bark, oak galls, Echinacea root, t-tree oil peppermint oil,cayenne pepper -massage in gums or use a water pick 4-6 dropper full to water

Supplement- molybdenum-needed by the dental enamel

Grape fruit; rind contains vitamin p = good for teeth and gums

MUCUS LACK (sjogren's syndrome)

Women with this problem produce too much estrogen, in relation to the amount of progesterone they make. Purchase progesterone cream and rub in on the belly.

Do not use store-bought salt, because it contains aluminum, which may damage the eyes.

For the eyes, add 1/4th tsp. Of table salt (or its equivalent in seawater) to one cup of water, bring it to a boil, and then let it set until it is tepid. Put some of this in the eyes every so often.

Take emulsified vitamin A, and use torula yeast. Black walnut husk tea may help.

MULTIPLE SCLEROSIS

Statistics cause: mercury fillings malnutrition, poor diet (meat, sugar, refined grains, rancid oils), stress, possible food allergies (dairy products, gluten), metal poisoning (lead, mercury etc. Chemicals poisoning, pesticides, vaccinations, toxins from bacteria or fungi in the body

-95% are found to have herpes symplex-6 -some have toxicity-some have heavy metal toxicity -mercury fillings in teeth may be a cause

Herbs-comfrey, chaparral, evening primrose, sarsaparilla, grape juice**,** echenesea , chaparral

Suma, gotu kola, kelp, chamomile, skullcap, valerian-black walnut 4 cap. 2x daily -sarsaparilla tea 3cups daily herbs high in plant sterols including licorice root, red raspberry leaf, black cohosh, squaw vine, ginseng and ginkgo.

Epson salt baths (2 hours or more) -Epson salt rub all over-then shower off-enema 2x daily-sunbaths daily - do not use heat therapy or wet sheet pack-1 lb. Pine needles + 1 lb. Pine cone + 1gallon water boil for 1 hour let cool for 12 hours strain and use 1 gallon per bathing provident in tolerance to heat, although mainly temporary

*Diet--*anti-inflammatory activity (for lupus, arthritis, multiple sclerosis, peptic ulcers, ulcerative colitis, crohn's, etc.): cabbage juice, olives, flaxseed and flaxseed oil (1-3 teaspoons, 1-3 times daily), celery (3 stalks pureed once or twice a day), nightshade free for 3 months trial (tomatoes, potatoes, eggplant, peppers, pimento, paprika), and gluten grains omitted (wheat, rye, barley, oats). Pineapple suppresses inflammation; so do apples and hawthorn berry tea.-100% raw -wheat germ oils

Avoid: -sugar, excess fat(proven to make problem worse) white flour, rancid oils, fried foods (they destroy the nerve cells)

Hyperbaric oxygen therapy has been used successfully in some other countries

Supplement: cold-pressed flaxseed oil is a source of linoleic acid (one teaspoonful per day) and borage seed oil, or oil of evening primrose for linoleic acid, can calm down an inflammatory reaction naturally.

It has been suggested that a deficiency of B-12 may be linked with multiple sclerosis (outside the U.S.).

NAIL PROBLEMS

A deficiency of protein or other nutrients can affect the nails. Finger and toe nails are composed almost entirely of protein. Some of the symptoms, followed by the deficient nutrient:

*Treatment-*Supply the indicated deficiencies, listed above, which apply to you. Eat a high-protein diet, including Brewer's yeast, calcium, silica, and, if necessary, hydrochloric acid.

Bending nails-rheumatoid arthritis

Bluish nails: chronic lung conditions (not enough oxygen).

Brittle nails: vitamin A, calcium/ iron deficiency, thyroid problems, kidney/ circulation problems

Chip or crack easily- nutritional/ mineral deficiency

Clubbed purple-rise upward and curl around the finger tips- lung/ liver/ colon/ heart

Curves downward and tip of nails- heart/ liver/ respiratory

Dry, brittle nails: protein, vitamin A, calcium, iron.

Excessive dryness, very rounded and *curved nail ends, and darkened nails:* vitamin b$_1$ deficiency.

Flat, spoon shaped- vitamin B12, anemia/ thyroid

Fragile and showing horizontal or

Fungus under nails: lack of lactobacillus in colon.

Grooves lengthwise- kidney, iron deficient/ aging

Half-moons absent: protein deficient

Hangnails: Protein, folic acid, and vitamin C/ fatty acid deficiencies.

Horizontal white lines- *sickle cell, heart disease, kidney failure, Hodgkin's*

Horizontal ridges- malnutrition, hormone disorder/ anemia

Pale nail beds*: anemia.

Poor nail growth: zinc deficiency.

Poor nail growth: zinc.

Splitting nails*: lack of hydrochloric acid, sulfur amino acid deficiency, calcium deficiency (tendency for arthritis).

Thick nails-improper circulation

Thin, flat, and even moon-shaped *(concave or spoon-shaped) nails*: iron deficiency.

Vertical red streaks-rheumatoid arthritis, high blood pressure/ psoriasis

Vertical ridges*: B vitamins. **Washboard ridges:** Iron, calcium, zinc deficiency.

White bands on the nails: protein deficiency.

White nails: liver disease, copper excess./ anemia

White spots: zinc deficiency, thyroid deficiency, and hydrochloric acid deficiency.

White moon area turns red- heart

White moon area turns slate blue-lung/ over exposure to silver

Yellow nails*: diabetes/ liver/ respiratory/ lymph

Symptoms: yellowish or greenish often accompanied with stunted growth and swelling of ankles and other parts of the body-cause: nutritional deficiencies -treatment: vitamin-e 800iu internally and apply to nail- do this for months

Treatment for fungus that causes nails to warp out of shape:

Black walnut tincture, plantain, t-tree paint to toenails x- 60-90 days

- Swedish bitters to area especially at night

-potassium permanganate (do not take internally)-will make toe nails brown soak feet x 1/2 hour in a warm solution 1:5,000 solution of potassium per... -dry feet- (dissolve slightly rounded tsp. Of the crystal in 8 oz. Water) - keep in dark bottle.-50-50 solution of vinegar and water x 15-20 minutes fungus nails

NASAL POLYPS	
Sniff goldenseal in tea form / cayenne/ pokeroot 2x daily, *blood root	

NAUSEA VOMITING	
Children-<u>can be a sign of Reye's syndrome (viral illness)</u>-withhold all food and fluids for 2 hours after vomiting *1 heaping tbsp. Charcoal* in 1/4 cup water or juice-use a straw or baby bottle *Herbal teas:* peppermint tea every 20 minutes, Ice chips -if vomit still give nothing for another hour -if vomiting ceases, give a little fluid after 6 hours -mashed bananas, potatoes, applesauce, rice, toast -return 24 hours later to regular diet with no (greasy food, spices, milk) -after feeding place infant on right side with folded towel on back (never on back -danger of choking) **Check**-bloody vomit- see cancer- stomach-sudden bout of vomit, sore throat, skin rash, -headache- see toxic shock **Sip plain hot water or hot** broth with some cayenne in it **Suck on lemon,** **Raw onion under each armpit** **Swedish bitters** compress to stomach **After vomit**-take spearmint or peppermint **Coffee enema***-effective-check iron deficiency-nausea after meals charcoal- **Hydrotherapy**-*hot fomentation* over the stomach with hot water bottle -ice pack against the back of the neck-ice pills, hot and cold compress over the stomach	**Powdered charcoal**+ ginger powder eliminates nausea **Herbs**: noni, 1/2 tsp peppermint + cayenne +ginger- safe for pregnancy-alfalfa mint tea, chamomile, fennel, dill, lemon balm, catnip, spearmint-peppermint - not safe for pregnancy, anise*, balm*,rosemary, basil* *Catnip or sweet balm* is also useful -willow bark- every 4 hours-little lobelia- 1 tsp to a cup of boiling water- take 1tsp every 15 minutes **Formula:** ginger root+ very small amount of licorice root and cayenne **Chemotherapy induced--**sweet basil **Headache due do nausea:** mild ginger tea compress to head **Nausea after meals:** check for iron deficiency B-6 200mg daily **Nervousness causing nausea:** catnip, hops, red clover **Pregnancy causing nausea:** goldenseal 3 cap, calcium 1000 mg daily, vitamin *<u>warning-large amount of peppermint tea causes miscarriage</u> **To induce vomiting:** -buckbean in large doses -lobelia• Use the treatments suggested for motion sickness; especially the charcoal and ginger root. It is said that powdered ginger root will definitely eliminate nausea.

NERVES	
Symptom: -sense of pins, tenderness, tingling, and loss of sensation to touch in the effected nerve area along with redness and swelling -weakness, paralysis, convulsions **Causes:**-symptom varies with cause-injury / infection/ disease (gout, diabetes, leukemia (etc.) To the nerve-lack of vitamin-b complex (especially thiamine)-a degenerative disease	**Nervous disorder and heart flutter:** formula -valerian root 1 part -caraway seed 1 part motherwort 2 part(mix and use 2 tbs. In 6 oz. Boiling water 2x daily) -apple cider 1/2 cup +cayenne 1tsp.+1 cup honey(take 1 tbsp. Every hour) **Nervous exhaustion:** b- complex vit

Fidgetiness:-fomentation to the abdomen followed by a hot abdominal pack

Empty colon- enema -neutral pail pour to spine

Herbs- St. John's wort - 1 oz. Each lady's, slippers and skullcap, 1/2 oz. Each wild yam, ginger, damania - pour 1 qt. Of boiling hot water over the herbs- cover let stand and cool-strain, sweeten to taste- drink 2-3 fl.oz. Every 3-4 hours

-valerian root, lobelia seed pods, passion flower herb, hops flowers, black cohosh root, blue cohosh root, skullcap , wild yam rhizome, rosehip tea

-lots of lemon -alfalfa mint tea 1 cups every 1 hour -aloe Vera - hyssop

-ladies slippers -feverfew -queen of the meadow

-juniper -strengthen the nerves throughout the entire body -blue vervain

-damania- toner over entire nervous system -gotu kola -ho-shou-wu-lyre leaved sage*, chamomile, valerian, dong quai, wood betony, passion flower, mistletoe and small amount of lobelia-noni

Irritability:-check for vitamin -b6 deficiency: valerian, passion flower, St. John's wort, chamomile, catnip, skullcap, oats, fit root, check for iron deficiency, dong quai-- provide tranquility for the whole nervous system

Swedish bitters-central nervous system- regulator-see guillain- barre-neurological weakness of arms, legs, **emotional stress :**St. John's wort, gotu kola, black cohosh, kava kava, b vitamins, ladies slippers, valerian **face-see myelitis-girdle pain:** check-niacin, phosphorus deficiency

Neuromuscular-check calcium, magnesium, manganese deficiency-check for calcium and magnesium deficiency

Neuralgia: passion flower=sedative

Neuritis: apply mild to moderate fomentations with revulsive over pain

Nutritional neuropathy=pins and needles start at tip of fingers and toes and spreads gradually due to alcoholism-treatment- b- vitamins, + minerals

Nervousness or mental illness: apply mild prolonged heat to body—neutral bath for one or more hours or warm fomentation to spine. Give catnip tea, one cup two or three times daily. Apply wet sheet pack. Give massage (total body or feet or back).

Nervous:-formula #1 -hops tea 5 tbsp. -cayenne 5 tbsp. - lobelia 5 tbsp.(mix in 1 quart of water - take 3-4 cups daily)

- formula #2 -lady slippers 1/2 part -valerian 2 part -mistletoe 1/2 part-hops 2 part -black cohosh 1/2 part -wood betony 1/2 part-lobelia 1/2 part-skullcap 3 part -goldenseal 1/4 part-mandrake 1 part-marjoram, valerian, prickly lettuce

Valerian root 1 tbsp., chamomile 1 tbsp. Basil, mint leaves, caraway seeds 1 tbs. Each mix 1 tbs. To a cup of boiling water- drink 2x daily

Sedative: common catalpa, common club moss* put one or two mild fomentations to back or to chest and abdomen. Leave each fomentation on for five minutes. Dry patient. Dress for bed.

Supplements:most important-- b- complex vitamin and thiamine copper supplements-keeps nerves calm-manganese- needed by the nerves, brewer's yeast, lecithin, kelp, dulse.-lecithin (from soy beans)- important for brain and entire nervous system

Tension: hawthorn*

Hydrotherapy-*1 lb. Pine needles* + 1 lb. Pine cone + 1gallon water boil for 1 hour let cool for 12 hours strain and use 1 gallon per bath-mint in bath tub- calms *(antispasmodic tincture)*

Alternate hot and cold to spine, hot foot bath brain and nerve

NIGHT SWEATS	
Check-hot flashes, caused by irregular thyroid activity. -Not enough air in a room can cause you to break out in an abnormal sweat **See-** tuberculosis, see Hodgkin's lymphoma *Hydrotherapy-*salt glow- before bed-take Epson salt baths(2 cups in tub) at night and hot/cold shower in morning-after night sweats are gone take 10 minutes cool bath in morning to tone the system	**Diet- fast 1 day each week-** on fruit and vegetable juice or distilled water- do not eat for 4 hours before bed• -avoid meat, salt, tobacco, and junk food. Drink 2 oz. Of green drink (whizzed up greens in pineapple or apple juice) every day. **Herbal:-** steep white oak bark or wild alum root in 1 qt. Water x 20 minutes and bathe in it -steep 1 tsp goldenseal in 1 pint water -drink 2 cups before bed -sage*-drink 2 oz. Green drink (whizzed up in pineapples or apple juice)-every day
NOSE	
Herbs-a=acute; sa=subacute; c=chronic; d=degenerative A-(runny nose, congested) mullein, cayenne, peppermint, rosehips Sa- (sinusitis, allergies) comfrey, myrrh, marshmallow, slippery elm C-(intestinal nasal clusters, polyps) goldenseal, myrrh, black walnut, capsicum D-(tumors) goldenseal, chaparral, burdock, Echinacea **Loss sense of smell**: zinc, check for tumor check for stroke **Nose bleed**:check-*Those with frequent nosebleeds should take extra iron.* High blood pressure. Avoid oral contraceptives. -vitamin-e oil in nose 7-10 days-white oak bark and bayberry sniff up nose then place cotton ball-goldenseal +1 pt. Boiling water-steep let cool and sniff up the nose -do same with witch hazel leaves, wild alum root, white oak bark-apply cold compress or pressure in back of neck -viamint-k in the diet-vitamin-c, calcium, mg, alfalfa, vitamin-e, iron, rutin- hot foot bath or hot leg pack-cold water spray to the bottom of the feet -put ice on hands, and elevate hands if possible to vertical position	**Nose postnasal drip -**Flush with saltwater and *gargle* with it.1/2 teaspoon of salt in about 8 ounces of warm water (the experts recommend only a third of a teaspoon, if you have high blood pressure). Suck it into your nostrils. 3 times a day for 5 days. -lemon and honey is helpful. **Herbs:***bee balm ,giant ragweed leave tea**dry powder made from- giant bird's nest** **Runny, stuffy nose:-** eucalyptus oil -chamomile, scotch pine, cayenne-1 part oil of spearmint + 1 part oil of peppermint mix with Vaseline and apply in nose with brush -1 oz. Witch hazel + 1/2 oz. Wild cherry bark + 1/2 oz. White oak bark -sniff the powder up the nose-witch hazel sniff up the nose or mix with Vaseline and place in the nose-take multivitamins, vitamin-a, steam bath -wet sheet pack -alternate compress to face **Hydrotherapy: -**ice bag to back of neck -short hot fomentations to face -hot foot bath/ leg pack -very hot nasal douche -elevate arms vertically **Relieve nasal congestion**—Alternate Compress to the face; Alternate Sponging or Compresses to the upper spine; Cold Foot Bath under running water if the extremities are cold.

OBESE

Check for the following:-hypothalamus, pineal, pituitary, thyroid, adrenal, pancreas imbalance-moon face- see Cushing's disease -see hypothyroidism

Exercise-Walking is always the best exercise it uses up to 120 calories per hour while actual jogging burns only 440 calories per hour.

-Swimming is done in cold water, triggers the body to store extra fat as protection against the cold. Swimming does not help one lose weight.

Formulas:uvaursi, bushu, juniper, couch grass, pipsissewa, lovage, celery**;** bladder wrack (make tea 1 tbs. In 10 oz. Water –drink 3 cups daily)**;**chickweed, garcinia cambogia

-mix: 2 tbs. Chickweed, 1 tbs. Irish moss, 1 tbs. Sassafras- place 2 tbs. In 10 oz. Of water. Drink 3 cups daily.

-plantain leaves -3 gm / psyllium seed 3 gm- in water 30 minutes before each meals causes increase weight loss-green tea helps you to lose weight

*Diet-*2 meal daily nothing to eat after 2 pm-spirulina 30 minutes before meals-reduces appetite-psyllium - 1tsp with juice water before each meal lead to loss of weight- drink 3 large glass water 3x daily on empty stomach 2 hour before meals or 1 hour after meal (to lose weight): all variety of fruits and juices, like grapefruit, orange, apple, pineapple, radish, tomato, lettuce.

Flaxseed 2 tsp daily- helps burn calories-24 hour fast /wk. All in one diet meal:1 cup rice milk, +1 cup soy milk,+ 1 cup fruit juice(apple, orange etc.,)+1 banana,+ 4 fresh strawberry (if available),+ 1 tsp black strap molasses,+1 tbs. Black cherry concentrate,+ 1tbs. Powdered green(barley, etc.) +1-2 tbs. Nutritional yeast,+ 1tbs flax oil---drink slowly

OSTEOPOROSIS

Avoidbrewer's yeast and tortilla yeast -eliminate milk -destroys bone-test have shown that high- protein diet causes calcium loss-eliminate meat- high phosphorus levels in meat-deprives the body of calcium-avoid "acid ash foods" (animal products, soda) -sugar contributes to osteoporosis

<u>Do not take</u> vitamin-d supplements-causes bone deterioration-(sun exposure a must) -smoking contributes to osteoporosis

Diet rich in bone forming minerals-tahini- for muscle cramps- osteoporosis preventive-calcium smoothie- ¼ bunch parsley +1 cup pineapple juice- blend till smooth. Drink daily.

Check hormone levels:-low testosterone in women is one cause-.take-tribulus

Formula: -comfrey root -4 part -horsetail grass -6 part -oat straw -3 part-lobelia -1 part -nettle -3 part, drink 4 cups of tea made from mixture daily-peach leaf tea 2 cups daily -take kelp tabs 3x daily and alfalfa tablets 2x daily-bring 2 cups of comfrey powder with 8 oz. Water to make tea

Supplements: -1,000-1,500 mg calcium daily (use dolomite calcium only)-800 iu. Vitamin e daily-magnesium 800 mg daily

Regular exercise a must-proven to increase the calcium level in bones

OVARY (salpingitis and ovaritis)

Hydrotherapy- Use hot and cold contrast sitz baths, to remove pelvic congestion and infection. Do this 3-4 times a day. Also apply alternate 2-3 minutes hot and 2-3 minutes ice cold compresses directly over the painful pelvic area.

Chronic form -hot vaginal irrigation twice daily; hot rectal irrigation once daily, if exudation in pelvis is extensive; pelvis massage. General tonic applications; general massage; sunbaths; out-of-door exposure

Acute form rest in bed; hot vaginal irrigation, twice daily; hot leg pack, hot pelvic pack; or hot footbath twice daily, followed by cold friction. During the first few days, ice bag over inflamed part, interrupted at intervals of 1-3 hours by fomentation for 15 minutes or hot and cold pelvic compress for 30 minutes; heat to limbs.

<u>Cautions</u>-avoid general cold applications and cold applications to the feet.

Herbal-(oophoritis, painful inflammation) licorice, false unicorn, black cohosh

(sluggishness) licorice, dong quai, black cohosh

(cystic tumors) chaparral, black cohosh, goldenseal

-Echinacea, goldenseal, black cohosh, black haw, and bearberry

Supplement-Vitamins A, C, E, and zinc are especially needed. Full vitamin/mineral supplement.

PAIN

TYPE OF PAIN

Abdomen

-*appendicitis*-pain and tenderness in lower right abdomen, vomiting, low grade fever, may have tenderness with pressure, pain quickly becomes severe, pain may be 1st felt over abdomen especially strong around the navel, coughing and deep breathing makes pain worse

-*Chromes*- abdominal pain -worse with food

-*cystitis*-pain in lower abdomen and back- with frequent urgent painful urination

-*diverticulitis*-abdominal, pain in left lower quadrant of abdomen, fever, chills

-*Ectopic pregnancy*- late menses with extreme abdominal pain

-*gallbladder*-severe pain in upper right abdomen, tender to pressure at lower edge of ribs on right side

-*gallstones*-constant pain in upper right abdominal-shoots in right or left shoulder region and radiates to back- pain can last 30 minutes to several hours

-*Gastroenteritis*-nausea, vomit, diarrhea, abdominal pain

-*Hernia*-pain, gas, abdomen distention, vomit

-*ileocecal valve syndrome* –right lower bowel tenderness

-*kidney stones*-initially an intermittent pain, dull, dragging, radiating from the upper back to the lower abdomen- usually increase with motion

-*pancreatitis*- pain can be from mild to sudden in upper abdomen

-*Peritonitis*-severe constant pain in the abdomen, fever

-*PID* (pelvic inflammatory disease)-female- abdomen pain, fever, vaginal infection

-*Pleurisy*- sudden severe pain with deep breathing in abdomen and stomach, cough or sneeze-in children pain in abdomen.

Back

-*Bright's*-lower back pain- see kidney,

Poultice: comfrey makes a very soothing compress

-lobelia, charcoal. - hops*over the stomach especially relieves pain -hyssop, mint, sage, Solomon's seal, burdock, comfrey

-*charcoal + smartweed boiled use tea, as fomentation

-charcoal poultice-cayenne poultice-with Vaseline wrap with saran -*plaster of Epson salt and grapefruit

Abdomen and back pain; -hot blanket pack

-large fomentation over effected area- followed by heating compress

Back-Lower back pain: -cayenne externally -thyme -lumbar-* plantain -exercise

-smoking has been linked to low back pain -flat feet linked to low back pain (wet feet make foot print on brown paper bag -if print is solid, no indents=flat feet) -maintain ideal body weight -8 minute ice massage (during the 1st 72 hours of the pain)

Cancer pain:paud'arco stops the pain of cancer**plaster of Epson salt and grapefruit, coffee enema

Coffee enema-*have known to relieve pain on hospice cancer patients

Eye pain: -soft flannel wet in hot salt water on eye* -charcoal poultice*-warm <u>not hot</u> fomentation over closed eyes

Intestinal pain: hot trunk pack **Muscle-Aching muscle:** -yellow sweet clover -selenium 100mg daily - proven to work

Neck pain:-ice pack on the back of neck wrap around towel

Perspiration-chills followed by profuse perspiration every 1-3 days, see malaria see TB/ aids-night sweat, see hyperthyroidism

Stomach: basil- stops cramps** hops poultice over stomach drink a glass of water every 10 minutes for 1 hour

Toothache: -mullein tea 2 cups -cayenne to area -catnip tea 2 cups

-*Constipation*-lower back pain, loss appetite, nausea, dull headache

-*endometriosis*- back, pelvic

-*prostate*- lower back, pelvic, groin

-*Small pox*-pain in back and limb

-*Yellow fever*-severe pains in head and down spine with fever and blood shot eyes

Bone-check phosphorus deficiency

Chest-Pleurisy- pain in chest when cough

Extremities-.ricket's/ osteomalasia- painful muscle spasms

Eyeball-dengue- pain around eyeball

Gallbladder inflammation-pain across chest and right upper abdomen

Knee, joint, jaw-knee-Osgood-shatter's syndrome- knee pain-Bursitis- joint pain-Temporomandibular joint syndrome- jaw pain

Leg, thigh, calf-Thrombosis-pain in legs (even at rest)-, pale, cold feet -arteries in intestines

Blocked= abdominal pain, vomit, fever-Phlebitis- pain to leg on movement- cordlike, swelling of vein-Sciatica- pain on back of thigh, the outer calf-Ankylosing spondylitis- back, leg, sacroiliac, hips, shoulder pain

Muscle-check magnesium deficiency

Nerve

-*Carpal tunnel syndrome*- thumb pain

-*Neuralgia*- shooting pain along a nerve

-*Raynaud's*-hand and feet extremely sensitive to cold

-*Tennis elbow*-tenderness and pain in elbow

-*Tic douloureuc*- face nerve pain thumb, elbow, hand, feet, toe, heel

Navel- check for parasites- pain around navel or appendicitis

Neck-check for parasites See meningitis-stiff neck-Polio- neck pain when bend neck down to chest, with fever

Pelvic-Ovaritis-salpingitis- pelvic pain felt on both sides

Prostate- lower back, pelvic, groin

-to area-- clove oil/sassafras oil/ oregano oil/ willow -mash plantain root put in cheek next to tooth -kerosene cotton in cavity -warm salt water wash –hot fomentation

Hydrotherapy-fomentations, moderately hot, for twenty minutes to the painful area.Revulsive for three changes to the painful area. Application of ice pack for fifteen to twenty minutes every two hours.

- Massage, either over the painful area or at a distance, as the feet, or head.

-hot tub bath with charcoal added to water bath additives-(mustard plaster)-fomentation-heating compress-muscle -joint- Russian steam bath

Formula: -1/2 cup cayenne -1/2 cup vegetable shortening - 1tbs eucalyptus oil /peppermint oil last in storage x 6 months (put in cloth or gauze x 3 hours)

Formula: -4 oz. Petroleum jelly-4 tbsp. Cayenne pepper -1-2 tsp peppermint oil or eucalyptus oil -1-2 tsp camphor oil (place on paper towel or gauze with ointment to skin and wrap with saran wrap)--x 24 hours

Herbs: - mullein -charcoal -smartweed -black cohosh -kava kava-white willow

-catnip-white willow-works like aspirin-reduces fever and pain-chaparral, noni

Compress of oat straw on painful area wild lettuce leaves- tea*

Supplement: -take - b- complex vitamin. -MSM topical lotion-selenium 100mg daily proven to relieve muscle pain

Pain liniment make from tinctures½ tsp. Clove-1 tsp. Cayenne-½ tsp. Peppermint-½ tsp rue-1tsp. Wintergreen-Arthritis- 8oz. Cold press peanut oil + 6 lemon juice- rub to area-or Vaseline / vegetable shortening+ cayenne +peppermint/ eucalyptus oil + camphor tsp. Or (bone/ cancer pain)-Vaseline 8oz. +7 tbsp. Cayenne (90,000hu) +3t ginger powder +peppermint oil 1tsp. +wintergreen oil 1tsp. Or 8 oz. Wintergreen oil + 8 oz. Witch hazel + 4-6 oz. Olive oil + 6-8 t 90,000 Hu cayenne

Rectum-rectal fissure -painful red, swelling at or near rectum **Toe-**See gout- big toe pain **Trunk-**Myelitis-pain encircling the trunk at the point where the disease is -*Spleen*- pain in the left side and extends up to the shoulders -*Mononucleosis*-pain severe pain in the middle of your left side that last 5 minutes or more, (go to ER) =splenic rupture **Chronic pain**-mustard plaster (2 tbs. Mustards+ 8 tbsp. Whole wheat flour- water to make a pie dough consistency- roll in plastic to ¼ inches thick- apply to chest and leave on till it starts to burn -clay, Swedish bitters- massage to area or take internally- 1 tbs. In a little warmwater- ankle injury- gives immediate relief	**Chia** –soak in warm water until thick and apply to affected area

PANCREATITIS

Symptoms: =a sudden attack of severe burning or stabbing pain in the upper abdomen--with vomit--worsen by moving--food worsen pain- pain may be mild if chronic may have excess gas, swelling and distension, muscle aches fevers, abdominal, hypertension, sweating, and abnormal fatty stools **Slippery elm enemas**. Cut the slippery elm bark into very small pieces, and put a large handful in 4 quarts of water. Simmer for 1-15 minutes, stirring frequently. Let it set, covered for 30 minutes. Strain and use it warm. Drink it and use in enemas. **Lobelia**-Place a heaping teaspoonful of lobelia in a cup of boiling water and let it steep for a half hour; then add a tablespoon of this lobelia tea to each cup of slippery elm tea, and drink. Also drink a cup an hour before each meal and before retiring. **Berries of eastern** red cedar: **herbs:-** charcoal-lobelia: tsp. Heaping, to 1 cup boiling water-steep x 1/2 hour add to 1 cup slippery elm tea and drink- nettle-papaya leaves-St. Benedict thistle -Echinacea, gentian root, goldenseal, cedar berries	**Herbs-a**=acute; sa=subacute; c=chronic; d=degenerative A-(infection) uvaursi, goldenseal, cayenne Sa (hypoglycemia) juniper, kelp, licorice root. Safflower C-(diabetes) blueberry leaves, juniper berry, goldenseal D-(degenerative stage) chaparral, Echinacea, elecampane, grapes, ginseng, pokeroot, licorice **Pancreas formula-** (All herbal aids give faster results in six days a week instead of seven, using the same day of the week of each week.) Hypoglycemia after six months or more of using two to three capsules or tablets three times in an day six days a week. They have had a glucose tolerance test with a clean bill of health on the pancreas area. Ingredients:*cedar berries-golden seal-uvaursi-cayenne-licorice root-mullein* *Diet-water* Fast and take only water until the acute symptoms subside. After coming off the fast because the acute phase is over, eat a low calorie, low fat diet. Low sugar diet. No alcoholic beverages, and also no caffeine

-licorice root-red clover -burdock root-milk this-tle-take Swedish bitters	**Very serious acute crisis**, give frequent hot steam pack fomentations to the abdomen. Give charcoal internally, and apply it as a poultice over the affected area.

PARASITE

These 3 will get rid of parasite + eggs if taken together wormwood, black walnut, common cloves from the clove tree. <u>Do not use wormwood during pregnancy.</u> **Ring worm**: cleanse bowel daily, 3 day citrus fast -Epson salt soaks, -garlic- cut a piece and bandage to area x 3 days-eat garlic -apple cider vinegar to area, sun bathe -vitamin-e oil + 1/2 tsp vitamin- a oil + 1/2 tsp lecithin, kelp +vitamin-e poultice -black motor oil x 7 days to area, -poke root bath - add 1 qtrs. Strong tea to bath -take vitamin- a, e and zinc, plantain and castor oil, t-tree -apple cider vinegar to area several times daily= part: castor oil, goldenseal, -rub area with borax and castor oil, black walnut extract, wormwood to area -take 2 chaparral or wormwood /golden seal caps daily -strong tea of = part plantain and yellow dock -scalp-wash hair with tar soap and borax-then steep 1tsp goldenseal+ 1/2 tsp myrrh in 1 pint of water and saturate hair- drink 1tsp goldenseal to 1 cup boiling water 2x daily -salve-= part burdock root, chaparral, wormwood + chickweed apply to area -lemon to area every few hours **Grapefruit tea** extract helps destroy parasites.	**Children**, crush garlic in milk and drink it throughout the day. Use a garlic enema every morning and put a garlic clove up the rectum before bedtime. Make sena tea, strain it, and add enough raisins to soak up the tea. Give the children a teaspoon of raisins 2-5 times a day. **Pinworms:** Eat 1-2 bitter melons each day for 7-10 days. Pumpkin seeds + garlic daily hot water enema with 3 tbsp. Salt, eat 1-2 bitter melons daily x 7-10 days-eat- 1-2 bitter melons each day for 7-10 days (available in Asian markets)-raisins soaked in Senna for children -infants-chamomile and mint teas **Clean the colon** with enemas and colonics. Take 2 per week for 4 weeks. **Hot water enema**, with 3 teaspoons of salt to a quart of water, may get rid of pinworms **Herbs:** clay-pumpkin seeds handful daily, heal all herb 2 cap. Daily, nettle 2 cap daily garlic 10 cap daily, ginger 2 cap daily, black walnut, wormwood, butternut, cascara gravada, goldenseal , MSM **Cut up two raw onions** and soak those 12 hours in 1 pint water; strain while squeezing out the juice. Drink a cup of this 3 times a day. Along with this, use garlic enemas. **Diatomaceous** earth capsules for 3 weeks, to get rid of your worms.

PERITONITIS

<u>**Bring to ER need immediate surgery or death**</u> **Symptoms:**(develops rapidly) -rigid, swollen abdomen, fever , nausea, vomit	**Post-surgery:** general treatment -warm bath-warm, wet packs to abdomen-castor oil packs-3-day carrot juice fast -tense abdominal muscles

Rapid pulse, sunken eyes, a pinched expression of the face -in severe cases dehydration and shock may occur

Hydrotherapy-<u>caution-</u> (avoid cold baths; instead use partial cold application, such as cold mitten friction and cold towel rub)

-Use warm, whole, baths or warm, wet, packs over the abdomen.

-Castor oil pack is also good.

If there is pain, take a slippery elm retention enema every morning

Herbs: bryonia, pleurisy root, aconite, slippery elm teas

on a regular basis tostrengthen- and helps rebuild

Diet-go on a 3-day carrot juice fast or a diet of oatmeal gruels, lentil and barley soup, and other potassium fruits and vegetables.

-During the inflammatory stage, avoid eating. Instead, drink as much slippery elm tea as possible, sipping it continually.

Once past critical stage: Once past the critical stage, drink comfrey root tea every 3-4 hours, along with Echinacea tablets

PHLEBITIS

Symptom: reddening cordlike swelling of the vein, pain to area on movement, slight fever, may appear red and swollen

Hydrotherapy-hot and cold showers morning and evening -hot- cold bath in tub

-very hot bath with 2 lb. Epson salt (no soap) for 20 minutes-then place in cold water for 10 seconds -walk in warm water mi-leg high-hot + cold foot bath (do at least 1 of the above therapy daily)-alternate hot and cold compresses to area

Take alternating hot and cold sitz baths or apply alternating hot and cold compresses.

Drink 2-3 quarts of water daily mix 3 lemons in the water

Herbal compress: yarrow, calendula flowers, St. John's wort,

-smear calendula ointment and Swedish bitters to area as a compress + do stinging nettle foot bath to improve circulation

Herbs:-gotu kola -butcher's broom -bilberry

If a swollen, painful vein does not disappear within 2 weeks, consult a physician. Include niacin in the diet. This B vitamin helps prevent clotting. Vitamin C helps strengthen the walls of veins and arteries. Vitamin E dilates blood vessels, reducing the formation of varicose veins and phlebitis.

Walk on wet sand: elevate legs at night, walk on early morning grass

Exercise-*do not massage the legs take a cleanser*

PLEURISY

Symptoms-pleural membrane inflamed, pain to chest when cough, sneeze , deep breathepleurisy can also occur at diaphragm surface- causes pain in abdomen and

Shoulders* in children pain is at the abdomen-

Cause: -too much cayenne on a daily basis proven to cause-pneumonia, bacteria, TB, damaged kidneys

Note do not jar the patients -jars and quick motion makes it worse

Pain- very hot fomentation for 10 minutes over the effected side- limit movement of lungs by tight bandage to chest- repeat every 2 hours

Cayenne and garlic mixture-1tbs every hour-1 tbs. Each hour of cayenne and garlic tea

Formula:- 1 tbs. Each of pleurisy root, yarrow, + pinch cayenne steep and-take a large swallow every hour*

Herbs:- pleurisy root *valuable take 4-6 every 2 hours +apply as a hot compress and give a high pleurisy root enema

Hydrotherapy- hot fomentations to upper back and chest x 1-2 hours -do 5 changes do notfollow with cold* - heating compress to chest (dry compress - wet sheet pack (sweating stage)	*Give hot herb teas*- of pleurisy root, yarrow, valerian, and buckthorn bark (add skullcap if the pain is severe) Too much during crisis)

PNEUMONIA

Symptom:-fever, chills, aching muscles, cough, sore throat, bloody sputum, enlarged lymph nodes in the neck, bloody sputum, pain in the chest, rapid difficult breathing and cyanosis **Poultice:** a-mash onions to chest area leave on for hours-1 part garlic + 1 part onion steamed with a little oil thicken with flaxseed /cornstarch- apply to chest in pillow case cover with heating pad **Diet**-*Only give liquids the first few days*. These should consist of fruit juices (diluted pineapple juice or orange juice) or lemon and water (without sugar), etc. Continue this until the high fever breaks. Then give strained vegetable broths, whole grains (best in dry form, so it will be chewed well). **Herbs:** -tea of- mullein, horehound, black berry, sage, white ash leaf, poplar bark, vervain -dandelion- excellent* -echenesia, kyolic garlic, goldenseal, fenugreek -astralagus- to boost immune -ginger- to fight the infection *Cough:* fenugreek tea **Cough**—fomentations every 3 hours; heating compress, changing every 15-30 minutes during the interval in between. Steam inhalation 15 minutes, every hour; sipping half a glass of hot water when inclined to cough; careful protection of neck and shoulders from chilling by contact with wet bed clothing. Keep shoulders covered.	**Small children:** -kyolic garlic (liquid)- the Japanese preparation-1 dropper full for infants and 1 tsp. 3x daily for older children **Fever**- only give liquids - diluted lemon without sugar-*after fever is gone*- give strained vegetable broth, whole grains (best in dry form), fresh carrot juice *Fever:* ginger , liquid kyolic garlic- 1 tsp 3x daily **Lung fever:** -compress on lungs -water freely on head-pain -cold compress to area- **Chest pain:** hot water bottle over chest <u>**Sore throat, asthma, bronchitis all lung problems, wheezing, fluids in lung**</u> -1/2 cup horseradish, ½ cup chopped onion, ½ cup chopped garlic, ½ tsp cayenne,1/3 tsp. Peppermint oil, 1 cup honey, ½ cup fructose-mix and take (1/2 tsp as needed-mix 1 cup boiled honey and ½ tsp. Peppermint oil, ½ tsp. Eucalyptus oil, 1/3 tsp. Clove oil, licorice root powder, and cayenne to taste *Hydrotherapy*-<u>do not use</u> cold full baths or anything equivalent -heating compress to chest -cold mitten friction -early stage - acute- dry chest pack -alternate compress **Keep bowels constantly cleansed** with enemas.

POISON

Immediatelly-charcoal-6 tbsp. **Non corrosive poisons**- induce vomiting (1 tsp. Salt in 2 cups of water)- drink it quickly- repeat 2-3 times if necessary-tickle throat wit finger **Take:** vitamin-c, pantothenic acid, beta carotene, Vitamin A helps the body discharge poisons	**Mercury:-sweating** helps excrete mercury -selenium (220mcg daily) eliminates it **MSG sensitivity:** vitamin b6 give 50 mg for at least 12 weeks (pregnant and lactating women should not take more than (100 mg of b6) **Mushroom:** -intense stomach pain immediately after eating it

Many poisons can be counteracted by taking an emetic to cause vomiting. (In the case of certain caustic poisons, vomiting is not the best.) *Put a teaspoon of salt in 2 cups of warm water and drink it quickly*. This will usually produce vomiting. Repeat a second or third time if necessary. Tickle the throat with a finger. After vomiting has occurred, induce more vomiting.

Herb-take goldenseal and myrrh every hour, Burdock, alfalfa, chaparral, dandelion, Echinacea, fennel, garlic, juniper, kelp, lobelia, and cayenne.

4 powerful antidotes: charcoal, garlic, vitamin-c, plantain

Alkali-strong alkali swallowed- swallow lemon and vinegar, drink white oak bark, alfalfa, oregano, or sweet basil **-gastric tube**- promote vomiting after 3-5 minutes (unless poisoning by acid, alkali, petroleum products or at risk for convulsions)- repeat this procedure 3-4 times -of charcoal and inducing vomiting .after

Aluminum poisoning: -calcium (1,500mg) and magnesium (700mg)- bind with aluminum and other metals -drink distilled water-tap water contains aluminum

Arsenic-onions, beans, legumes, and garlic to obtain sulfur. Only drink distilled water. Drink plenty of fruit and vegetable juices.

Caustic material (Clorox etc.)-do not induce vomiting- will cause damage first *swallow soda, chalk, lime and water, milk, or vegetable oil- to neutralize* the acid then induce vomiting

Chemical-cleansing fast for 2- days every month

Food poisoning: Pain, vomiting, cramping, weakness, diarrhea, dizziness.

Symptoms occur quickly, 1-4 hours after eating the contaminated substance. They can last for a few hours or a few days.

-*take*:-6 charcoal tabs, 2 garlics 3 x daily- teas of- wormwood- 3x daily, cloves-burdock root tea -clean colon with enema-induce vomit with lobelia

-take acidophilus every few days to encourage growth of good bacteria's which produces

-quickly empty the stomach- take an emetic to cause vomiting/ tickle throat, 1 tsp. Salt in 2 cups warm water and drink quickly keep repeating it until vomit-take to the emergency room-take to the emergency room

-if the fly amanita- after emptying the stomach a shot of atropine must be given

-*swallow lots of charcoal in water*-(2 tbsp. In a glass of water

Poison ivy: -run hot water as hot as possible to area)- this wash off the oils

-bathe in ocean water, sap--baking powder to area,

-place to area- Epson salt, calcium powder

-plantain poultice

-jewel weed leaf- poultice* ranks at the top for cure (neutralizes the poison)- rub plant to area or make ice cube of the tea and apply to area-bloodroot, Echinacea, goldenseal, lobelia, myrrh, chicory

-2 parts yellow dock + Echinacea 2 parts + 1 part chaparral put in capsule and take 2 cap every 2 hours-wash area with lemon juice or apple cider vinegar

-*blister:* aloe -apply powdered calcium to area-stops itch-apply vitamin-e oil to area

-*Banana peels*, rubbed directly on the area, bring relief for as long as 4 hours.

-*itching:* Wash lemon juice over the area, and then pat dry. -apply poultice of = part- comfrey root, slippery elm, witch hazel, aloe Vera,

-apply a tea made of 50-50 white oak bark and lime water.

Radiation poisoning /chemo

-*Clay*

-*herbs: maitake extract*- take 2-3 drops daily-ginger - nausea

Glutamine (5,000-15,000mg daily) - protects the digestive tract

-.antioxidants vit- mineral therapy-Siberian ginseng- 200mg 3-6x daily

- astralagus- 1,500 mg daily-green tea (500mg) herb/- take several cups daily

b- vitamin-goldenseal extract-every 4 hours for 24 hours	- umeboshi- for nausea and vomiting-= Japanese tea
-use enemas to clean the colon-induce vomiting-with lobelia - or place finger in throat	Astralagus, Echinacea, goldenseal, burdock root, chaparral, dandelion, milk thistle, red clover, birch, suma
-apply fomentations over the stomach while keeping the feet warm	*-if you are not obtaining enough calcium your body* - will absorb more-paint iodine on top of your foot or inside of your thigh to protect you
-give 2 tbsp. Castor oil-no food for 24 hours except for increase water intake	*-Supplements:* -panthotenic acid (200mg) -inositol (100mg) -lecithin granules (1tbsp.)
Glass bits of glass- eat lots of soft bread-	-b- complex -vitamin-e (400-800 iu.) -calcium (2,000- 5,000mg) -potassium (5,500mg)-mag-
Poisoning food	nesium (750mg) -zinc (50mg) -coenzyme q10 (100mg) -dulse/ kelp (1,000mg)-aloe Vera has
Take 6 charcoal tablets immediately, and again in 6 hours. Drink lots of good water (distilled is best).	been found to reduce radioactivity -chlorella and spirulina-protects against ultra violet radiation-cleanse blood stream
Heavy metal poisoning do hair analysis to deter-mine- treatment =chelation	

PREMENSTRUAL SYNDROME (PMS)

Herbs which may help reduce the pain of cramps: rosemary, black haw, cramp bark, red raspberry, kava kava, and angelica. Dong quai, false unicorn root, fennel seed, squaw vine, blessed thistle, and sarsaparilla root. They	**Hydrotherapy**-Use warm sitz baths, heating pad, or hot water bottle for cramps. This draws the healing blood and relaxes muscles.
-Selenium is an antioxidant and helps prevent menstrual cramps.	**Supplement**-Vitamin E, Vitamin B$_6$ (50-150 mg daily, especially during the 10 days preceding menstruation

PROSTATE

Herbs-a=acute; sa=subacute; c=chronic; d=degenerative	**Enema-high charcoal** and water enema helps the healing process. Use 1 cup of hot water to 1 tea-spoon of powdered charcoal. Allow it to remain
A-(inflammation) goldenseal, queen of the mead-ow, pumpkin seed, comfrey	as long as possible. **Hydrotherapy**- acute condi-tion, take hot sitz baths daily and add chamo-mile tea to the water;
Sa-(enlargement) buchu leaves, yarrow, chaparral	Helpful is a short cold bath**Cautions**—When pain is present, avoid general cold baths, cold
C-(hernia) comfrey, fenugreek, willow, marsh-mallow, cayenne	Sitz Baths, Cold Footbaths, and chilling of feet. Absolute sexual continence is essential.
D-(degenerative stage) goldenseal, myrrh, Echinacea	**Supplement**-Treat it with zinc (50 mg, three times a day), essential fatty acids (flaxseed oil,
Tea- 1 oz. Each saw palmetto, damania, got kola – simmer in 2 pt. H2o till1 pt. Is left –1 cup 3 times daily after meals--or-tea- 1 oz. Each couch grass, buchu, marshmallow+1 1/2 pints water-simmer for 15 min. 1cup q4h-or-tea-1 oz. Couch grass+ 1 oz. Buchu+ 1 oz. Marshmallow in 1 ½ pt. H20 simmer for 15 min. -1 cup 4 times daily	1 teaspoon, three times a day), and a high-fiber diet which includes pumpkin seeds and alfalfa. Vitamin A (as beta-carotene, 300,000 IU a day), vitamin C to bowel tolerance, chlorophyll (as

Urinary blockage -buchu tea, one to two quarts per day -hot and cold alternating tubs

Herbal: -saw palmetto -pumpkin seed -200 mg daily/ 1/4 cup raw seeds daily -licorice-pygeum (50mg of the bark extract, 2x daily) -stinging nettle (2-3 tsp. Of extract daily)-Echinacea, goldenseal, horsetail combine with hydrangea helps contract the prostate -cayenne

Formula: -mix equal part- corn silk, buchu leaves, parsley, saw palmetto berries, kelp, pumpkin seeds, plus a pinch of cayenne

alfalfa), selenium (250 mcg, three times a day), amino acids (alanine, glycine, and glutamic acid; 5 grams each, daily for 90 days), and cranberry juice (2 pints a day).

1/2 cup pumpkin seeds in a blender, open one capsule of saw palmetto and pour in blender, add a few drops of licorice extract- blend until smooth (a few drops of flax oil may be added) -keep refrigerated -spread on bread -eat a couple of tbsp. Daily (make 2 day batch only at a time

PSORIASIS

Swimming in the ocean,

Check-allergy foods. Beware of milk and wheat. It may be well to exclude them for 6 months, even if they may appear harmless. Avoid fats

Supplement-Vitamins A, B complex, C, and D all help the skin and appear to be of help in

Itching-a cold-water bath, perhaps with a cup or so of vinegar added, is very helpful. Another help is ice. Put some in a plastic sack and hold on the area.

Herbs nettle, Echinacea, oat straw, shave grass, horsetail grass

PULSE

For-increase rate- do hot foot bath-increase heart above 120 - ice bag to heart

Pulse and respiration too fast- immerse both hands in very cold water (55 f.)

RASH-See skin section	
RAYNAUD'S	
When an attack occurs, immerse the body part in warm (not hot) water, no warmer than 90° F. During an attack, without realizing it, one's skin can more easily burn. Massaging the hands and fingers every evening helps reduce the severity of the attacks **Herbs** include garlic, ginkgo, biloba extract, and pau d'arco.	**Take** vitamin E (80-1,200 unites per day), unsaturated fatty acids alone (wheat germ oil, etc.), tryptophan. Take calcium (2,000 mg daily) and magnesium (1,000 mg daily). Get enough iron in your diet. Zinc is also very helpful in this condition. -Sprinkle a small amount of cayenne on your food, to increase circulation.
RECTAL ITCHING	
Check for pin worms **Warm (not hot) tea** bag of goldenseal may be applied to the area for up to a half hour, to relieve itching Or rub wheat germ oil	**Hot sitz bath daily**. After the bath, apply lemon juice to the area with a piece of cotton **Squeeze lemon in rectum** **Take pulse tests**(see allergy section) to check food allergies

SCIATICA

Check calcium deficiency

Topical: compress with mistletoe team, massage onion to area

Add 2 cups of salt to a boiling quart of water. Apply warm with a cloth to the area until relief comes.

Supplement: b- complex, calcium, vitamin. D, E, B12

Herbs: burdock, nettle*, dang quai , willow bark, wintergreen-mix 2 tbsp. Grated ginger +3 tbs. Sesame oil + 1 tsp. Lemon juice- rub to area

Exercises: Rub the limb.do stretching exercises- do each 3 times 2-3 times daily

Hydrotherapy-*bath*:-2 cups baking soda in hot water daily

-Apply heat in the form of hot fomentations, 3 times a day, omitting any use of ice or cold water. After each application of heat, rub the limb to increase circulation

SEIZURES

Check for: magnesium deficiency-check colon impaction, constipation in the transverse colon-give catnip enema (child or adult)

-The artificial sweetener aspartame (nutrasweet) has been linked to seizures.

-check improper functioning of ileoconduit valve- cause toxins in blood to brain -*check parasite- use garlic*

Antispasmodic tincture One-half ounce cayenne pepper and 1 ounce of each of the following herbs: skullcap, skunk cabbage root or seed, gum myrrh, lobelia seed (or the plant if the seed is not obtainable), and black cohosh root.

Mix each of the above together while dry and put into a large-mouth jar. Add 1 pint pure grain alcohol of 70-100 proof. Eighty proof Vodka works fine because it is tasteless.

(An alternative to alcohol is to, instead, use 1 pint of apple cider vinegar. Store in the same manner.)

Let this stand for 10-14 days, tightly covered, and shake well, daily.

Then strain it through a very fine cloth and squeeze out all you can. Store it in a tightly capped bottle. Also put some into a small dropper bottle.

In a crisis, it is given in 8-10 drop doses. Squirted into the mouth or taken in a tbsp. Of water. (If stored in vinegar, give in teaspoonful doses, not drops. Its effects are not quite as rapid.) Released

When attack is threatened—colonic twice daily; copious water drinking; neutral pack; ice to head; rest in bed. Seizure may sometimes be averted by placing the part in cold water.

After attack—rest; cold to head; cold mitten friction or cold towel rub; half bath; revulsive douche to legs; and percussion douche to spine.

Colon cleanse- parasite treatment

Enemas or colonics

If the bowels do not move each day, take a lemon enema (juice of 2 lemons in 2 quarts water) before going to bed that night

If parasites- use garlic- if constipated- use catnip enema

Supplement: -vitamin-B6 100mg 2x daily -B-complex daily-calcium (2000mg) daily and. 1000mg daily-E 1000iu daily -chromium (75-100 mcg, 3x daily)deficiency of manganese- take supplement

-<u>caution-</u>do not give large dose of folic acid will increase seizure activity

Formula:-honey -1 cup; -cayenne -1/2 tsp; -horseradish - 1/2 cup chopped-yarrow - 1 tbsp.; -clove tincture - 1/3 tsp; -myrrh - 1tsp; -goldenseal -1 tbsp.-garlic -1/2 chopped; -ginger -1/3 tsp

Herbs: <u>avoid sage</u>

-catnip, skullcap, peony-take 2 cups of valerian root tea every 2 hours-rue, black cohosh, valerian, vervain, peppermint, chamomile, wild cherry

from clenched lockjaw by a small application of antispasmodic tincture.

When the case is severe, especially with an infant, the tincture can be rubbed onto the chest, neck, and between the shoulders. Place 2-3 drops in the mouth, and wash down with teaspoon doses of warm water while the person is kept in bed. If necessary, repeat every 1-2 hours.

Infant (*put them in a tub of 95f. Or mustard water bath 85f.*)

-produce vomit (put finger down throat) -fever (tepid or cool bath)

-*gums hot and swollen*- give cold water and rub ice to gums

-*immediately* give laxative herbs -keep body warm

-fast on fruit juice, water or nervine herb teas until symptoms disappear

-lobelia tincture should be rubbed well to neck, chest, and between shoulders

-The bowels should be emptied immediately with an enema.

- Fast on fruit juices, water, or nervine herb teas (listed below) until all symptoms subside. Keep the body warm.

-After this, rest in bed, absolutely quiet; give careful diagnosis without disturbing him.

-check food allergy (pulse test) (see allergy section)

bark, goldenseal, and little cayenne -after seizure must rest in bed-give weak chamomile tea in small doses several times a day

Formula -passion flower, hyssop, and skullcap are very good for epilepsy. The formula for one day's dosage is: 2 tabs. Of passion flower, and 2 tabs. Of skullcap. 2 tabs. Of hyssop, put the teas into a quart to a quart and a half of boiling water and steep for half an hour. Make up fresh every day. Half the formula used in half the quantity of water can be given to a child. *For severe cases the formula may be doubled for either children or adults.*

Preventing seizures—Do not eat soft bread; better yet, do not eat any bread. You may find that you should not eat mush either.

SENSES

Zinc supplements :proven to heighten sense of smell, taste, sight-30-60mg zinc- 3x/d

Taste: -copper supplements -heightens sense of taste -b-vitamin supplements plus-zinc 30mg daily for several weeks then reduce to 15mg daily

Pins and needles, loss of sensation:-peripheral nerves damage due to lack of b- complex vitamins (increase risk in alcoholics)-treatment-vitamin-mineral supplements- B vitamins B1 (1000mg)

SHINGLES

If the shingles appear on the forehead, tip of the nose, or near the eyes, contact ophthalmologist. Such cases can lead to blindness.

Clay bath or spread over skin fever treatment for 2 days

Put apple cider vinegar on it daily. Take hot baths 2-3 times a week. Take a starch bath (one cup of cornstarch or colloidal oatmeal) into a hot tub. Colloidal oatmeal is powdered,

Calamine or other calcium preparation on them

Charcoal compress- grind fresh green leaves and apply to area vitamin E, aloe, honey, peppermint oil **DMSO-**apply licorice to area-cold cloth to area-apply cayenne to area (it works so well to block pain)= FDA approved cream-ice block massage x 20 minutes 2-3x daily	**Take goldenseal or myrrh** tea (1/2 tsp. To a **Massive doses of vitamins C** (1,000 mg 3 times a day and 200 mg 5-6 times a day), cup) or 3 capsules

SINUSITIS

Humidifier **Heat lamp** (60 watts) over sinus-incandescent lamp **Two cups Epsom Salts**. Add a teaspoon peppermint oil. Hold a cotton cloth by the edges and dip it in the water. Twist it to remove excess water. Then just hold it over the sinuses. **Sniff** up some weak goldenseal tea- **Formula sinus & lung-** Brigham tea, horseradish, and cayenne. For immediate relief of sinus pressure due to cold or allergies, use 20 drops (1/4 teaspoon) in 1/4 cup of hot water. May be taken every 1/2 hour **Herbs:** -6 charcoal tab between meals 2x daily-garlic tea - boil 4 cups water -add crushed garlic cloves relieves **supplements:** -vitamin-c (500mg) every 2 hours until the problem goes away-NAC (nacetylcystein)- 500mg 2x daily **Take a short fast on** citrus juices, vegetable juices, and herb teas	**Compress:** -hot application -see sinus pack -strong peppermint tea -cold application- with hot foot bath- hot foot bath-alternate hot cold application -2x daily apply a heating pad to your chest- **Alternate hot /cold compress**-hot Epson salt packs (add salt till water becomes thick, place small wrung out towel over face , and place a dry towel to keep heat in, leave on till cool (rub peppermint oil to nose prior)-revulsive to face. **Mix 1 tsp. Of salt with 2 cups** warm water. Pour it into a small glass; and, holding back your head, sniff it up into one nostril (as you pinch the other one closed). Repeat for the other side. **Sinus pack: -**make a weak goldenseal tea and sniff through nostril-peppermint oil 1 tsp +Epson salt 5 cups +clove oil 1/2 tsp+ water 1 qt.(mix and boil---dip face in hot mixture 3x daily or use compress)

SKIN DISORDERS

HERBAL-a=acute; sa=subacute; c=chronic; d=degenerative A(irritation, inflammation) chickweed, plantain, comfrey, goldenseal Sa-(dry) red clover, oat straw, shave grass C_ (psoriasis) nettle, Echinacea, oat straw, shave grass, horsetail grass D-(degenerative stage) chaparral, Echinacea, goldenseal **SKIN SYMPTOM (DEFICIENCY)+** TREATMENTS (EFA=essential fatty acids)	**ITCH:-** goldenseal 1 part + vit-e oil in honey -mix and apply -oatmeal bath - 1 lb. Of cooked oatmeal - apply in cloth place in tub of water -2tbs. Vinegar to bath water-take- yarrow, violet, marjoram -mix = amount -marshmallow root, fennel seed, dried plantain, violet leaves , steep, strain drink 1 qt. Daily -lemon juice-slippery elm ointment- 1/2 cup olive oil +3 tbs. Slippery elm heat for 5 min. +add 2 tbs. Cocoa butter when melted cook for 10 min.- strain through cheese cloth-pour in tight fit jar- refrigerate till firm (last for 2 months)-wet salt

-_adrenal exhaustion_ (increase tanning at folds of skin, elbows, knees: black freckles)-all B vitamins, pantothenic acid, vitamin V; all minerals, digestive enzymes, allergic testing, avoid sweets

-_arterial spiders_ (on face, neck , chest)-antioxidants, bioflavonoids, glucosamine, calcium

-_bedsores-_ vitamin C,E

-_blisters-_ vitamin E

-_brown discolor_ around small joints- vitamin B 12

-_brown skin spots-_ antioxidants (weak liver)

-_bruised areas easily under skin-_vitamin C, bioflavonoids, rutin, grape seed extract, alkalizer, glucosamine

-_dermatitis on infants-with inflamed_ pustules around body openings- Vitamin B6, zinc,biotin Scrotum, vulva- vitamin B2

-_dry skin-_ (Vitamin A,C, EFA)

-_eczema, skin ulcers-_ vitamin C, B2, B6 zinc, magnesium, EFA, allergic test, cleanse

-_eczema, infantile-_ zinc, EPA, vitamin B6

-_eczema scaly around nose, ears,-Edema-_ vitamin B6, C, zinc, magnesium, (avoid salt)

-_eyes- greasy dermatitis_ around eyes, nose- vitamin B6, zinc

-_Fingers, numb, stiff, swellings_ (Raynaud's) vitamin B6, B1, niacin, antioxidants, magnesium, calcium, EFA

-_fish like scales_ (ichthyosis)- Vitamin A, retinoic acid, MSM

-_folds of skin red and infected-_ niacin

-_fungus infection_ (athlete's foot, ringworm)-b- vitamins, need colon cleanse, apply t-tree oil

-_Gangrene-_vitamin E, B1, C, magnesium chloride

-_goose pimple like skin_ (keratosis)- Vitamin A internally and externally

-_greasy skin eruptions-_ vitamin B2

-_hardening and swelling of skin_ (scleroderma)- vitamin A, E, C, magnesium chloride, MSM, (parasite cleanse, t-tree oil packs)

-_Heat rash-_vitamin C

-_hot flashes-_ Vitamin E, boron, magnesium, calcium –use wild yam cream

-boil 6 onions x 15-30 minutes and apply liquid to skin -oxalis leaves make into a paste and apply-itching of genital- wild comfrey

-soda alkaline bath-ice water compress ,oatmeal compress-anise oil to area

KERATOSIS (SHARKSKIN) • Take vitamin A supplementation. This should be 25,000 units per day, for children, or 30,000 units per day, for adults. However, keep in mind that vitamin A can be dangerous; since it is an oil-soluble vitamin; it is normally stored quite well by the body. Many experts recommend never taking over 50,000 units a day and only for a limited period of time.

Increase zinc to 50 mg, three times a day, and essential fatty acids to 5 gm, three times a day-deficiency of vitamin a and zinc-take 25,000 units vit-a daily for a limited time only -take zinc 15 mg daily -essential fatty acids 5 gm 3x daily

LEUKODERMA (Vitiligo) —This is a loss of skin color -causes - _thyroid, b-complex deficiency_

B complex supplementation, plus emphasis on two special B vitamins: Para-amino benzoic acid (PABA, 100 mg four times a day) and pantothenic acid. PABA injections may be needed. Also be sure and take hydrochloric acid if it is needed. • Other helpful nutrients include vitamins A, B complex, B12, zinc, and copper.

Symptom-lack of skin color- white patches surrounded with dark border-

Take: PABA, pantothenic acid, mg, zinc and copper - b12 (1000mcg every 2weeks) produces normal skin color in 8 months. *folic acid (1-`10 mg daily) *b-complex vit. - l-phenylalanine (50mg per kg. Wt.)-combine with

.ultraviolet radiotherapy- ultra violet lamp/taning beds

Herb: khella-120- 160 mg daily, St. John's wort

Take hydrochloric acid if needed-stop taking if burning sensation in stomach

MOLES: if mottled look and flat and larger than the top of pencil eraser(get it checked for cancer) -if mole turns blue, white or red, or begins to bleed --have it checked for cancer-milkweed,

-infection-(boils, cold sores, impetigo etc.)- vitamin C, A, B6, EFA, zinc, magnesium chloride (hot Epson salt packs, t-tree oil or propolis rubs)

-insect bite sensitivity- vitamin B1, C, alkalizer, calcium, bicarbonate rub/ bath

-itching- vitamin B, C, alkalizer, bicarbonate rubs, allergy test

-jaundice- vitamin A, C. E, B12, magnesium, lecithin, zinc, - use blue light therapy, treat gallbladder and liver

-oily skin- white heads- Vitamin B2

-pale skin- biotin, folic acid, vitamin B6, iron (see anemia)

-purplish, blue black areas- vitamin C, B2, bioflavonoids

-rash- allergic test, alkalizers, vitamin C, calcium

-red skin on pressure areas- zinc, vitamin B6

-Red-brown/ or dark red spots- manganese

-Rosacea –(red around part of face)- vitamin B2

-scar tissue- vitamin E, MSM (internally and externally), camphorated oil rub

-shingles- vitamin B12, A, C, E, B, lysine, zinc oxide lotion

-Skin cancer- vitamin B6, A, PABA, bioflavonoids, antioxidants, chlorophyll, propolis, and zinc. (take a piece of raw bruised garlic as big as the cancer area apply with a bandage for 3 days only)

-Sunlight over sensitivity- vitamin B6, zinc, PABA, beta-carotene, antioxidants, bioflavonoids, alkalizer

-sun exposure causered-brown symmetrical discoloration, later ulceration-niacin/ niacinamide (folic acid)

-swelling (example face)- vitamin B6, B12, magnesium , zinc

-vaginal itch- vitamin B2, C, E (see candida, no synthetic underwear)

-warts, moles- Vitamin A, C, E

-wheals (urticarial)- vitamin C, B6 zinc, (alkalizer, allergic testing)

piece of garlic to area- x 3 days -change daily-to remove a mole suspected to have cancer- place slice of garlic on it nightly for 2-3 nights

ERYTHROMELALGIA (NECROSIS) —A skin neurosis, accompanied by burning and throbbing .Let the patient rest. Elevate the affected part. Place a cold compress on it, and change this every 20-30 minutes. Apply graduated tonic frictions, such as the wet hand rub, the cold mitten friction, or the cold towel rub.

OILY SKIN: -apply herb teas of- yarrow, sage, or peppermint-mud mask (white or rose colored

PORES ENLARGED- mash half an avocado and put it on your face. Leave it there until it dries, and then wipe it off with water. Avocado has essential oils.

-To reduce puffiness under your eyes, place cool slices of cucumber over them for 10 minutes. .

PRICKLY HEAT:(SKIN FEELS HOT AND PRICKLY) -wash 2x daily with mild soap

-after a bath use 1/2 tsp cider vinegar in a glass of water -take vitamin-c orally more than 1000mg daily

PSORIASIS:-apply Swedish bitters, vit-e 5000iu, vit-a 150,000 iu., lecithin 4 tbs. Mix in 16 oz. Add to unpasteurized milk and apply at night and wash off in morning

Aloe internally uses juice or gel 1-2 t, 1-2 times per day. Externally, use 2 times per day as a juice or ointment.

Apply -cream containing capsicum -vit- d3 cream -rub mashed avocado to area -chamomile- apply a tea to dry and flaky area-licorice / sarsaparilla -as tea and apply to area-take-combine in tea and take- milk thistle seed, oregano grape root, dandelion root, yellow dock and garlic-works in 1-3 months-angelica

Make strong decoction of 8 oz. Garlic juice and glycerin +1 pint of burdock seeds- mix -saturate cotton and place on area -change 2-3x daily and drink 1 tsp 3-4x daily

Cleanse-take slippery elm/ American yellow, saffron to heal the bowel wall, drinks lots of water-1/2 tsp slippery elm powder to 1 cup of warm

-_white skin patches_-PABA, vitamin B6, zinc, pantothenic acid

-_wrinkles or aging_- vitamin A, C, E, EFA, bioflavonoids

ALL SKIN ERUPTIONS:- herbs to take: red clover, burdock, Echinacea, goldenseal, yellow dock, red root, jojoba*figwort _jojoba pine sap good for skin_ <u>do cleanse</u>

-zinc supplement excellent proven treatment-flax oil (vitamin-F) reduces and heals

INFLAMED SURFACES, SKIN ERUPTIONS, CANCEROUS SORES, ITCHING DERMATITIS, AND HIVES: Drink burdock seed tea (as a diaphoretic to open skin pores and glands from the inside), and wash the affected parts with a strong decoction 2 or more times daily (more often for local eruptions). Apply chickweed ointment, or a chickweed bath

ADHESIONS:=scar tissues from a surgical site

-massage tiger balm 1 inch around area in a circular motion till it is healed do this 5 minutes daily-until the site is healed about 2-3 weeks (do not pull on or across the surgical site)

AGE SPOTS/ LIVER SPOTS: -lemon oil, -take gotu kola, burdock, milk thistle, comfrey root tea -aloe gel-dandelion- sap of the crushed stem-slice of red onion-fresh pineapple/ lemon-juice-watercress leaves to skin-take nutritional supplements-vitamin-E 1200 units daily-A (beta carotene)

B- complex –B2 vitamin-take grapefruit seed extract daily

BLISTERS:-ice-peach pit tea-dandelion stems-add methione, lysine in diet-apply lavender oil to area-2-3 times daily -pain and itching- ice to area-apply the white sap of dandelion stems daily and apply bandage till healed

BLOTCHES-cause = impure blood--- liver toxic- cause- microorganism

BROWN SKIN SPOTS: + **aloe Vera-said** to decrease or remove with 2 times a day application using the juice or gel. It takes several months-aloe Vera poison ivy to many eczemas. Simply rub the liquid or gel directly onto the area of

water let stand for 15 minutes- do not eat for 30 minutes- do this for 10 days then every other day till psoriasis disappear-take - lecithin 3 x daily -5 days a week-American saffron- 1/4 tsp saffron to 1 cups boiling water- let stand x 15 minutes-drink it for 5 days (stop if excessive urination or bladder irritation)

Itchy - oatmeal in warm water or bath like warm bath of 1 cup apple cider vinegar

Skin cracked from scratching -2/3 cups rolled oats,1/3 cups cornstarch, 1lb.baking soda

PUSTULES: root- kamala*

RASH: apply cool compresses to area for 10 minute-comfrey/ chamomile tea to area-compress of calcium water (1tsp. Calcium glutamate water in 1 cup of water)-oatmeal water compress -chamomile tea wash area -poultice--dandelion+ yellow dock+ chaparral and plantain

Heat rash- take a soda alkaline bath in 95-98 sit in tub and continuously pour water over you for 30-60 minutes- then stand in tub and partially drip dry - then pat self-dry or put 1-2 cups of peppermint leaves in tub of cool water (immerse the mint for 3-5 minutes)- soak in tub for 5-10 minutes

Rash/ infections of skin:-garlic ear oil 1 drop 2x daily-proven to treat fungus better than drugs (1 cup chopped garlic. Cover with 2 cups cold pressed olive oil. Let sit for 7 days, shake daily. Strain oil into dark glass bottle with a top . Store in fridge -potatoes grate and mix with slippery elm for a paste and apply to area

SCALLING- soda alkaline bath 15 minutes to 1 hour Neutral Alkaline Bath daily for 15 minutes to 1 hour

-cause- stress, nutritional deficiency (especially vitamin-a and biotin)

-treatment- vitamin.-C, A, B-complex -eat gluten free diet -colloidal silver

SCARS:-scargo -vitamin-e -lavender oil -aloe Vera -comfrey poultice

-_badly healed scars_- marigold* vitamin-e 400iu prevents (topically) also take internally dermatitis -psoriasis and eczematous rashes: internally use juice or gel 1-2 t, 1-2 times per day. Externally, use 2 times per day as a juice or ointment

BRUISING EASY (Ecchymosis) (kidney and liver disorders. Anemia)

Alfalfa tablets and a good vitamin-mineral supplement 2-3 times a day. Vitamin K. Vitamin D is another natural clotting factor.

Herbs -burdock, aloe Vera, cayenne, kelp, and white oak bark. Garlic, alfalfa, and rose hips

BRUISING (Contusions)

Ice pack on the bruised area and keep it there for 30 minutes. Later apply a poultice of greens (fresh or dry), oatmeal, wheat bran, comfrey, or charcoal. Pulverize the charcoal, tie it in a cloth, wet it in warm water, and lay it over the bruise for several hours. Repeat until it is better.

CANCER OF SKIN: -piece of garlic to area and tape x 3 days **;** aloe Vera juice 2-4 times per day for months

CHAPPED SKIN:-olive oil + lemon oil -take vitamin-e, vitamin-a supplement-water and aloe Vera mist or essential oils to water mist -mashed avocado; facial-oatmeal bath

COMPLEXION:-onion

CHILBLAINS—Alternate Foot Bath; Revulsive Douche to feet; Alternate Douche; Hot Foot Bath, followed by Foot Bath under flowing (cold) water; foot pack.

DERMATITIS: mixture of clay and glycerin

-goldenseal compress or poultice is made by putting 1 teaspoon of goldenseal leaves or 1/4 teaspoon of powdered root in 1 cup of water. Bring it almost to a boil. Allow to set off the fire for 15 minutes. Dip a folded linen or paper towel in the tea to saturate but not drip. Place directly on the skin. .

Supplements: -vitamin-B complex 300 mg daily -vitamin-b6 100 mg 2x daily

-kelp 5 tab 2x daily -vitamin-E 800-1000 iu. Daily -zinc 60-100 mg daily

-vitamin-A +d 25,000 iu. 2x daily

-apply lavender oil on skin or mix it with aloe Vera gel and apply to prevent scarring-comfrey poultice accelerates healing along with the above mentioned treatment

Can combine aloe Vera and vitamin e to form a salve

SPOTS: -lemon

SORES, ABSCESSES, PUS: vitamin-e, c, b-complex poultice- slippery elm bark and lobelia poultice, honey to area, goldenseal, myrrh, comfrey as paste

STRETCH MARKS: aloe Vera itself or mixed with vitamin varicose veins.

SWEATING- (inactive skin- not sweating)- hot cold baths, cleanse

-take Bromelin -400-500 mg 3x daily on an empty stomach

-tea of chamomile, comfrey, mugwort, dill, oregano- drink and apply externally-ginger-ice to area-arnica-(mountain daisy)- widely used for sport injury-corn silk- used in china for years to reduce swelling-dandelion -make a tea of chamomile, comfrey, white oak bark, mugwort, dill or oregano drink and apply to area

SWEATING FEET—Revulsive Douche to feet, with extremes in temperature as great as possible; alternate hot and cold Foot Bath, Heating Compress to feet during the night, with Cold Mitten Friction to the feet, in the morning on rising

SWELLING-Take Bromelin (which is fresh pineapple enzyme), either in tablet form or in fresh pineapple juice.

-Make a tea out of chamomile, comfrey, white oak bark, mugwort, dill, or oregano.

-Drink it and apply it externally to the swelling.

A contrast (hot and cold) bath or shower may help relieve it. Cold water alone may do it. A raw potato poultice over the area

ULCERS:(POULTICES-)-German chamomile, marigold, arnica, cliff rose, snake root, witch hazel, red clover, carrot and beet juice, burdock, cayenne, yellow dock root -diluted t-tree oil excellent*

Herbs: -charcoal 1 tsp 2x daily in water-comfrey root 3 cap 3x daily- red clover 5 cap 2x daily -myrrh 3 cap 2x daily -lecithin 1 tsp 3x daily- MSM- good for skin, bones, nails, joints, cartilage teeth,

Hydrotherapy: - baking soda bath,*neutral bath --itch or dry

DRY LIPS from toothpaste:-brush teeth with baking soda-lip balm, lavender oil (30 drops)+ sandalwood oil(15 drops)+2 oz. Cocoa butter or flaxseed oil

DRY SKIN chafing: check for essential fatty acid deficiency, underactive thyroid

-vitamin- a (if you are taking it dry skin=1st sign of overdose)

-take flax oil and wheat germ oil (cut of all other oils from diet, vitamin-each, b-complex, zinc-ripe avocado or ripe banana to skin- wait 15 min. And rinse

-add 2-3 drops of lavender oil to warm water and apply warm compress to face-short sweating bath

-Pour 2 cups of oatmeal, ground to a fine powder, into a bathtub of warm water.

ECZEMA: a goldenseal compress or poultice is made by putting 1 teaspoon of goldenseal leaves or 1/4 teaspoon of powdered root in 1 cup of water. Bring it almost to a boil. Allow to set off the fire for 15 minutes. Dip a folded linen or paper towel in the tea to saturate but not drip. Place directly on the skin.

Bath: -*soda alkaline bath -oatmeal bath (use colloidal oatmeal from pharmacy) -charcoal baths-

Herb -zinc supplement -proven to clear eczema -lemon -red clover, dandelion, plantain, chickweed, burdock, - comfrey, dandelion, plantain -yarrow, strawberry leaves-chamomile, gingko bilboa, licorice root ,witch hazel-root, yarrow, strawberry leaves -make tea and apply

Apply:-mix juniper wood oil with yellow wax and apply-instead of soap use oatmeal tied in cloth -dip in water-mix goldenseal root powder+ vit-e oil-

-simmer several peach pits and wash area with the tea and apply compress also

-goldenseal, myrrh and comfrey into a paste can heal almost an sore

Supplement:

- vitamin B5 (panthotenic acid)-protects against skin cancer, eczema, skin cancer -vitamin-B17 (laetrile, nitrilosides)-PABA-selenium good for all skin problems-flax oil-vitamin-E

*Healing salve:*2 cups cold pressed olive oil, 2 cups of dry calendula flowers, 1 cup fresh plantain leaves, simmer them for 4 hours in a double boiler- strain oil

Add 1 oz. Bee's wax, preserve with 1 tsp. Vitamin e oil, add 6-10 drops lavender oil pour into glass or hard plastic containers, add comfrey for bones

GANGLION:(GANGLION CYST)-symptom-hard bump develop on wrist or back of hand, sometimes on the foot-varies in size from a pea to plum-causes-develops near joint= sac of jelly-like painless-compress of- witch hazel or white oak bark tea, take antibiotic herbs

GENITALS-Swollen Testicles, Burning and Itching Bathe the area with a strong decoction of chickweed and apply chickweed ointment.

GRAFTS:-paraffin bath

HEAT RASH: soda alkaline bath

HEMATOMA: compresses of Solomon's seal-makes skin more beautiful tincture

Of arnica, kidney vetch- excellent, sanicle

HEMORRHOIDS and Rectal Cancer: Bathe the area 2-3 times daily with the decoction, infusion, or diluted tincture (as warm as possible), then apply chickweed ointment.

HIVES:(problem linked with candida)to terminate recurring hives do a long fast 1-3 days in length ,use enemas during the fast

Apply--jewelweed tea to area -ginger-simmer 1/2 lb. In 1 gallon water take hot bath after the bath sponge of with chamomile tea = excellent-apply chickweed ointment-calcium glutamate paste -apply milk, calamine, milk of magnesia

Steep: burdock root + yarrow+ yellow dock in 1 pint water x 1/2 hour -strain add 1 lb. Cocoa fat and keep boiling until it is a salve-*figwort, evening primrose oil -rosemary oil to area -aloe Vera -evening primrose to area -red clover and goldenseal compress -infants-mix-primrose oil and vit- b6-

Tea formula- 1oz each of yellow dock +chickweed + burdock + ½ oz. Buckthorn bark+ 2 qt. H2o- simmer drink three times daily with meals

Hydrotherapy:-alternate hot and cold compress-avoid wheat gluten

ERUPTIONS:/SORES; aloe Vera, t-tree, chamomile tea, *peach powdered bark or leaves *rosemary oil to area, alkaline soda bath (1ounce solution to 1 gallon of water) / oatmeal bath If *dry,* not irritable, give prolonged Neutral Bath. If *scaly,* alkaline bath (soda bath or oatmeal bath). If *moist* and irritable, cool evaporating compress moistened with soda solution (1 oz. To 1 gal.). If skin is *thickened,* as in chronic eczema, Hot or Alternate (hot and cold) Spray Douche or Compress for 10-15 minutes, 3 times a day. If *extensively damaged* skin (as in pemphigus, confluent smallpox, bad burns), the Continuous Neutral Full Bath until the skin is healed

ERYSIPELAS: symptoms- red, discolored, blisters, swelling, fever-face

Treatment-cold compress to area-use no soap- wash with a saturated solution of boric acid-herbs: plantain, yellow dock, chickweed, burdock root, chamomile, mullein, yarrow- dissolved any one in 1 qt. Water dip cloth and tap area (do not rub) (chickweed is the best one)

Formula: =part-gum myrrh, Echinacea, witch hazel, goldenseal- mix

1tbs to 1 pint of water---steep x 1/2 hour-strain and apply with cotton

Raw cranberry poultice-applied cold cover area with 1/4 inch thick of raw grated potatoes

No matter how bad the pain and swelling, make a decoction from a handful or two of fresh chickweed. Bathe the surface every 1/2 hour and apply chickweed ointment (the pain and swelling will be gone in a few hours).

Take - chamomile, wild oregano, rue, parsley, basil, Echinacea, fennel, yarrow -burdock tea 3-4xdaily -drink chickweed tea and apply chickweed ointment

Bath -baking soda/ Epson salt bath -aloe Vera to area -*immediate* help-soda alkaline bath -apply chickweed ointment and take chickweed baths -hot bath with 1 lb. Of baking soda or Epson salt (draws out toxins

Supplement - vitamin-c (2000mg every 4 hours), vitamin-b-complex, calcium, b6,b12, take - hydrochloric acid with meals- quercetin 2x daily

IMPETIGO CONTAGIOSA: *contagious*-this is a common childhood disease(2-8 year olds) need isolation-cause- streptococci infection-symptom- redness followed by a blister-like swellings followed by a honey colored crusted lesion which heals slowly with loss of skin color (may last for months) -most common effected area is face and extremities

-lesions itch-treatment:- remove the crust - bath area in soapy or 1/4th strength peroxide with water -firmly adherent crust apply warm compresses-centralized lesions- starch poultice -keep nails short -to prevent spreading -change pillow cases and bed sheets daily (boil linens to prevent spreading to other children) -do not swim -expose area to sunlight -Venus maidenhair fern* -compress of boric acid, comfrey, goldenseal, Echinacea -place garlic oil-diet: no oils or sugar-charcoal poultice

.hydrotherapy: -five changes of hot (3min.) And cold (30 sec.) Compress

-if lymph nodes are involved do hot tub bath keeping head cool

Supplements: -multivitamins, vitamin-a, c

ERYTHEMA—Cool evaporating compress or irrigating compress (explained just above); neutral compress.	
FRECKLES: root- kamala**watercress- apply leaves to area	
INACTIVE SKIN—Sweating process, followed by a cold	
INFECTED/ PAINFULL: pine sap to area	
INTERTRIGO-(skin eruption from body parts rubbing together)	
-due to yeast and fungus growth obese, diabetes-apply starch to add dryness, (never talcum/ baby powder) eat garlic and acidophilus , -apply chamomile tea, aloe Vera gel, t-tree oil use cotton clothing	
SPLEEN	
Symptom- moderate swelling and pain in the lymphatic tissue, chills, high fever, severe pain develops in the left side and extend to the shoulder, deep general flush with raised borders in the affected areas, skin becomes hot and dry, excessive thirst-cause =streptococcal infection of lymph glands specially spleen-hot- cold fomentation to painful area do this 3-4x daily until pain is over-liniment- mix 2oz. Powdered myrrh + 1 oz. Powdered goldenseal + 1/2 oz.	**Hydrotherapy-** see wet sheet pack (heating stage) **Herbs:** bistort root, gum weed
Cayenne- put in 1 qt. 70 % alcohol shake daily--- good for all swelling and pain	
-keep bowels open	
A=acute; sa=subacute; c=chronic; d=degenerative	
A-(inflamed) blue violet, Echinacea, goldenseal	
Sa-(sluggish) capsicum, blue violet, Echinacea	
C-(chronically inflamed) Echinacea, goldenseal, blue violet	
D-(degenerative stage) goldenseal, Echinacea, chaparral	
STOMACH	
Herbal-a=acute; sa=subacute; c=chronic; d=degenerative	**Cramps/ pain:** *lobelia tincture , *bee balm -charcoal 1 tbs. + olive oil 1 tbs. – mix and take 1-2 x daily
A-(ulcers, indigestion) peppermint, celery, alfalfa, papaya, goldenseal , capsicum, slippery elm	

Sa-(stomach flu) goldenseal, blue violet, myrrh, geranium

C-(HCL imbalance) rue, wild cherry, celery, licorice root

D-(degenerative stage) alfalfa, comfrey, chaparral

Acid-achlorhydria (insufficient stomach acid):- symptoms- burping, belching and bloating- lemon juice before meals-English bitters (gentian lutea) -betaine HCL (75-250mg) 15 minutes before meals-avoid gum -

Herbs- gentian and milfoil increase stomach juice, angelica, St. Benedict thistle, or sweet flag, pineapple-*hydrotherapy*- cold mitten friction before breakfast, cold douche spray over stomach 3-4 hours after meals, hot abdominal packs small cold enema- retained, do it 3-4 hours after eating ice bag over stomach cold enema before breakfast-drink 1/3 glass of cold water half an hour before meals

Acid-excess stomach acid:-eat smaller meals- take vitamin- mineral supplements

Avoid -cold baths, cold douche over stomach and spine

-hydrotherapy-hot douche over spine opposite the stomach -hot douche over stomach, hot emersion bath (105 f.) For 15 minutes painful digestion-hot fomentation 1 hour after eating for 15 min. Followed with heating compress to be worn till next meal

Delicate stomach: false unicorn***Formula -stomach tonic: formulas*-mix 3 gm. Wormwood + 2 gm. Peppermint + 1gm garden sage, steep in 1 cup boiling water- strain-cool- take 1 tsp. In water 1/2 hour before mealsmix 3/4 tsp. European centaury +1/2 tsp. Buckbean+ 1/4 tspjuniper berries- infuse in 1 pt. Water- take 1 tsp. In water 1/2 before mealsmix 1 part each buckbean, ceataury, germander, and blessed thistle- infuse at a rate of 1 tsp of combined herbs to a cup boiling water ---take 1- 2 tbs. Between meals

Gaseous distended abdomen: hot enema- followed by small cool enema / cold colonic- cold abdominal compress (change hourly)

Nervous stomach: yellow sweet- clover, chamomile

Phlegm in the stomach: *chicory

STOOL

Babies-Diarrhea, impaired growth in babies- copper deficiency

Black stool- see cancer- stomach

Black/ red stool- parasites

Blood-Diarrhea, blood in anus, sometimes with mucus- see polyps (colon)

Bloody diarrhea, mucus, gas, pain- see colitis

Bloody stool- see colon cancer, bleeding, parasites

Bulky, pale, foul feces=malabsorption, check for deficiency for b12/ iron, cystic fibrosis, celiac, lactose intolerance, pancreatitis-check for parasites-Irritable bowel syndrome- pencil like stool

Confusion-Diarrhea, confusion- see beriberi, pellagra

Diarrhea- see constipation

Fever with diarrhea= serious infection

Light colored stool- see hepatitis

Light colored stool-see hepatitis, jaundice

Loose, watery, often with bloody, mucus- dysentery

Loose-Mild morning loose bowels- see sprue

Offensive- see typhoid

Pale-Diarrhea, pale and/ light yellow, foul- smelling stools float- see celiac

White/ pale stool= disease of liver-Burning, stinging when passing stool, possible bleeding of rectum= (rectal fissure) **Chronic diarrhea**, chronic rectal bleeding, pale, bulky fatty stools floats chrome's	**Sudden diarrhea**, confusion, rash, headache, vomit- toxic shock **White curd** like masses in stool and stool is thin- see cholera

STREP-THROAT

Grape fruit seed extract: put on throat- gargle and swallow **Gargle** goldenseal tea- 1cup 3-4x daily, gargle colloidal silver, salt water gargle- increase circulation to area **Hydrotherapy**: ice collar, cold application, place a heating compress to the throat, hot foot bath along with hot and cold compress to throat heating compress to neck	**Antibiotics**-goldenseal, echenesia, garlic are fenugreek and comfrey loosen the mucus **Broth diet** for 3 days .vitamin, a, selenium, zinc. Catnip tea **Enemas** put peppermint tea helps settle the stomach, charcoal in mouth several times daily

SYPHILIS

Symptoms: a sore in the genitals, sores in the mouth or anus. A rash, patchy and flaking tissue, sore throat, fever **Hydrotherapy**:-salt glow-steam bath **Formula**: -yellow dock -2 tsp -bayberry-2 tsp -barberry -2 tsp-blue violet -5 tsp-red clover -7tsp -prickly ash berries -4 tsp -bugleweed -1 tsp-bloodroot -2 tsp-bitter root -1tsp (mix and take 5 caps 2x daily). *Formula:* mix 2 tbs. Each of; buckthorn bark, uvaursi, burdock root, red clover blossoms, oregano grape, blue flag root prickly ash berries + 1 tsp. Bloodroot-steep 1 heaping tsp. In a cup boiling water x 1/2 hour -drink 4 cups daily- 1 hour before meals and at bedtime*take them for at least -1 year vitamin-c 4000mg daily.	**Herbs**-Echinacea, yellow dock, burdock root, bayberry bark. Goldenseal, pau d'arco, Echinacea, sassafras, suma **Eruptions**: bathe area with 1 tsp. Each of goldenseal and myrrh **Sores:** -lemon juice / vinegar to area--daily x 5 days -muriatic acid / nitric acid to sores x few minute then rinse-then apply glycerin-gotu kola **Swollen glands in the groin:** -lemon juice rub to area -poultice of ground roasted poke root / slippery elm and strontium leaves 2x daily- *Sweat treatments:* and salt glow **High enemas daily:** **Pain and tension:** hops tea **Treatment for 2 years**

TESTICLE

Herbal-a=acute; sa=subacute; c=chronic; d=degenerative	**Testicle inflammation, acute**
A-(epididymitis) goldenseal garlic, willow, Echinacea, myrrh	Rest in bed; elevation of scrotum upon a tense broad band of cloth, placed about the thighs close to hips; Hot Pelvic Pack or Hot Hip Pack with Cold Compress over genitals, every 3 hours. During intervals, Compress at 60^0 F. Over perineum, genitals, and over stomach, with heat to feet. Tepid Enema, twice daily; Cold Mitten Friction or Cold Towel Rub, twice a day; prolonged Neutral Bath or Neutral Pack to control temperature
Sa-(retention/ morbid matter) saw palmetto, cayenne, goldenseal	
C-(impotency) damania, false unicorn ginseng	
D-(VD, tissue degeneration) chaparral, Echinacea, goldenseal, garlic, myrrh	
Undescended testicles see gland for formula for	**Testicular atrophy**
Hydrotherapy:- hot pelvic pack with cold compress over genitals every 3 hours- during interval-compress 60 degrees over perineum, genitals, stomach with heat to the feet- tepid enema- 2x daily-cold mitten friction or cold towel rub 2x daily- prolonged neutral bath	Results at times after mumps causes less sexual drive and possible feminization
	Vitamin/ mineral supplements zinc 30mg 3x daily, saw palmetto and ginseng. Eat a nutritious diet, plus a full range of vitamin/mineral supplementation.
	Take zinc (50 mg, three times a day).
	–herbs-saw palmetto and ginseng.

THROAT

EPIGLOTITIS- <u>Urgent</u> fever, severe sore throat dysphagia, bluish skin/lips **ESOPHAGITIS** Chest pain, occur only post swallow or eat	**SORE THROAT** -Swelling/ lumps sides of neck, fever/ sore throat/ flu symptoms
	STREP THROAT -Swelling/ lumps sides of neck, fever/ sore throat/ flu symptoms *,no runny nose*

THROMBOSIS

Symptom: pain even at rest go to the emergency room, intestinal artery block= stomach pain, fever, vomit	**Herbs:** -garlic, mistletoe, lemon tree, sesame, linden -smear calendula ointment to area and bitters as a compress to area and do stinging nettle foot baths to improve circulation
Hydrotherapy: continuous application of moist heat for 20 of every 24 hours are often recommended (covering the entire extremity)	

THRUSH

If your baby has thrush, which you can determine from white spots on the sides of the mouth, a white tongue, or soreness during nursing, you can try several remedies. Give raspberry tea in a bottle. *Ingredients*: oak bark-golden seal root-garlic-comfrey-myrrh-capsicum	**Infant thrush** -swab area with baking soda solution-blend 1 peanut size garlic in 1 cup of water and swab area-simmer 5 bay leaves in 2 cups water, let cool, 2x daily apply to mouth with a dropper
	Persimmon- tea from the inner bark ,cleanse mouth with every feeding

Baking soda wipe mouth 4x daily **Garlic solution** swab several times daily blend 1 peanut size clove in 1 cup water	**Simmer 5 bay leaves** in 2 cups water x 20 minutes- strain- cool apply to mouth With dropper 2x daily- refrigerate last x2 days

THYROID

Herbal-a=acute; sa=subacute; c=chronic; d=degenerative

A-(hyperthyroidism) kelp, dulse

Sa- (hypothyroidism) kelp, dulse, goldenseal, black cohosh, myrrh, bayberry

C-(goiter) kelp, Iceland / Irish moss

D-(degenerative stage) kelp, Irish moss, dulse

Avoid- chlorinated water , fluorinated water, toothpaste(they block entrance of iodine in the thyroid)- electric blanket, nitrates

Treatment: -liquid iodine- 3 drops 3x daily/ paint an area 3x3 inches on thigh it will be absorbed in 24 hours if deficient, myxedema up to 30-50 .kelp dulse/ Norwegian kelp -about 4-6 tabs 3x daily

-sarsaparilla- 5 cap 2x daily .black cohosh 2 cap daily / 1 cup tea daily

-licorice -6 cap / 1 cup tea 2x daily.

-Coconut oil- restores hormones- 1oz. In am and 1 oz.in pm. Wheat grass- 7 tab daily.

-Olive oil 1 tbsp. Daily.

-Molasses 1 tbsp. 2x daily.

-Lecithin 1 tsp 2x daily.

-Gentian with or without cayenne,

-saw palmetto .

-logo's solution (by prescription only). -Amino acid 500mg 3x daily.

-Black walnut 2 capsules 2x daily for 2 weeks.

-Swedish bitters , clay are excellent take by mouth and apply poultice

Enema:-coffee enema 1x weekly .see anemia drink formula

Diet: go on a raw juice fast the raw foods for 2-4 weeks

-radishes has been used in Russia to treat both types of thyroid problems

Herbs: -gentian tend to normalize function of the thyroid (take it alone / combine it with cayenne, kelp, and saw palmetto) -take 1 kelp tablet daily

Hydrotherapy- see- Russian steam bath -steam bath / salt glow 3x weekly

Treatment for goiter: enlargement of thyroid gland-Epson salt compress around neck all night x 10 nights

-white oak bark tea compress around neck'-put 2 hot fomentation around neck for 4 minutes each and 1 cold compress for 4 minutes alternate this cycle x 1 hour- then 5- 10 minutes neck exercises poultice of ground almonds completely around neck all night x 3- 10 nights-

-apply black walnut extract as paint on the throat all night x 3- 10 nights

-calendula: take 1/2 droperful of extract and apply the herb compress to neck 2x daily x 1 months

-mix burdock root + olive oil apply to neck

-*To eliminate goiter (an enlarged thyroid gland):* Follow the above program; and then, after the 2-4 weeks, do one or more of the following four neck applications: Put an Epsom salt compress on the neck every night, and leave it on all night for 10 nights. Use a compress of white oak bark tea over the goiter for better results. Put two hot fomentations around the neck, for 4 minutes each and one cold compress for 4 minutes. Continue alternating this for an hour. Then spend 5-10 minutes doing exercises with the neck in various positions. Put a poultice of ground-up almonds completely around the neck and leave it on all night, for 3-10 nights. This is especially good for harder, more fibrous, goiters.

Supplements: niacin 100mg 2x daily-vitamin- b 12 1000mcg daily-vitamin-c 500 mg daily -olive oil 1 tsp. Daily -black strap molasses 1tbs.

-fresh juice of green walnuts (especially the husk)- doubles level of thyroxin -decoction of green walnuts-made by boiling them 20 minutes, boosted thyroxin at least 30% -remain oil-free, salt-free, sugar-free diet -eat oats and bananas daily	2x daily -wheat grass 7 tabs. Daily -lecithin 1 tsp. 2x daily - vitamin a- necessary for iodine to properly absorb - the b-vitamins work together to nourish the thyroid-b6 helps the thyroid use its iodine effectively-b12 helps the thyroid use its iodine works properly

TONGUE

Pellagra-red inflamed-sprue-smooth -anemia - pernicious- sore tongue **Acidity**:-pallid tongue- pale without color with white fur **Alkalinity**: -deep red tongue **Aseptic poisoning**:(blood poisoning)-dirty coating, tongue=dark in color, with brownish to black fur **Beefy enlarge tongue-**pantothenic acid deficiency **Blisters**- apply Swedish bitters **Blue veins under tongue** (cracked lips and corner of mouth) vitamin b2, b6, folic acid deficiency. **Brownish coat typhoid**-tongue and lips **Burning sore-** vitamin b2, b6, b12, niacin deficiency **Diphtheria-** greyish coat in mouth, and throat **Edema/ tooth marks on tongue-** niacin/ niacinamide deficiency **Elongated tongue=**, pointed, reddened at the tip, red at the edges-treatment= increase water intake hot foot bath Stomach and bowel disease + body effected **Mouth cancer**- persistent sores in tongue	**Paralysis** Tongue or throat: -cayenne 1 tsp -apple cider vinegar 2tbs-sage tea 1/2 pint -sea salt 2tbs -honey 2 tbsp. (gargle with above mixture 4-12x daily)-cold compress at night over spine **Red at tip or edges-** b6 deficiency **Scarlet fever-** tongue coated white **Slick tongue** -general weakness and run down feeling- b12, folic acid deficiency **Sore tongue-** iron deficiency Stomach irritation with blood detrimitation= (excess blood in the intestines) **White painless patches**: Tongue -see teeth and gum Tongue red, sore and inflamed: vitamin-b deficiency, allergies **Yellowish, moist fur-** intestine (small intestine): weak will be uniformly coated from base to tip **Yellowish, brown coated-**liver-gallbladder problems

TONSILLITIS

Cause: - tonsillitis is due to accumulation of toxins **Babies**- use blackstrap molasses in formulas instead of sugar to regulate bowels ½ cup raisins + ½ cup apple added to pure water. Small amounts of cascara sagrada and ginger can help to regulate bowels	**Herbs:** -if no herbs -paint tonsils with glycerin -babies give prune juice -mullein, blackberry, bistort, raspberry, white oak bark -sage, slippery elm, red root, white pine bark needle , -blood root*adenoids or tonsils -calamint*3x daily give red clover, sassafras + burdock**gargle daily (several x with goldenseal) take echenesea and myrrh -dissolve charcoal in the mouth several times daily-goldenseal, Echinacea, garlic

10 day cleanse-citrus-eliminate cow's milk, white flour products, wheat possible allergy)-lemon/ lime juice in warm water with honey and ginger will help the cleansing process

Adenoids:*butternut bark

Diet: -eat nothing but oranges and grapefruit for 3 days -1/2 lemon every day for 3 days-drink raw cabbage -apple juice

Fever, pain ,swelling: -1/4 tsp. Lobelia extract (swallowed every 2 hours) **fevers:** -catnip tea enema

Gargle: -charcoal-goldenseal tea, and drink -1 cup 3-4 x daily)-cayenne-lemon -salt water-t-tree diluted -Echinacea –myrrh

Mucus: -fenugreek and comfrey

Pain inflamed: ice pack to neck

Soaks to neck: -Epson salt

Hydrotherapy:-heating compress to throat-hot foot bath along with 5 minutes hot cloth and 5 minutes cold cloth to throat- finish with - see heating compress to throat, daily sponge bath, daily sunshine

Sore throat: -1 drop of t-tree to tongue and rub on neck-kerosene on outside of neck-then cover with flannel-gargle cayenne/lemon-colloidal silver

Cold mitten friction then immediately UT him to bed-drink plenty of fluids

Supplement:-high intake of vitamin-c, vitamin-a, selenium and zinc

TUBERCULOSIS

Symptoms: -coughing, general fatigue, night sweats, and low-grade fevers, loss of appetite-cough starts non-productive and later becomes very productive -person loses weight and sputum becomes bloody

Causes: -mycrobacterium tuberculosis -it is contagious (travels by air)

Hydrotherapy: -graduated cold application -sun-baths -cold air baths-outdoor exercise and living

Sweating treatments (don't be surprise if boils develop = toxins exiting)

-*heating chest pack* which begins cold was applied on retiring at night and removed in the morning.

Live in elevation regions - not damp lowlands

Cough: ginger, licorice, slippery elm, marshmallow, mullein -honey 1 cup + peppermint oil ½ tsp. + cayenne ½ tsp. Lemon juice 4 oz. Mix and take 1 tsp. 3x daily

Formula mix 2 oz. Each of dandelion root, yellow dock root, bittersweet, and stlinga root with American ivy (orVirginia creeping bark or only its twigs) - simmer in 3 qt. Water reduce to 2 qt.-strain. Sweeten with honey, let cool- take 1 tbs. 3x daily

Diet: 85% raw, green drink 2x daily -juice- 8-12 oz. Carrot + alfalfa 2 tbs. + parsley 2tbs.+spinash 2 oz. + watercress 2 oz. Comfrey powder 1 tbs. + onion 2 oz. Garlic 2 oz. (mix–drink 8 oz. 3x daily)

Herbs: -drink lemon water 3-4 lemons per qt. Water daily -pineapple juice or fresh whole 6 oz. 3x daily -gotu kola, herb Robert -Echinacea –take 2- 450mg cap 3x daily-garlic daily -licorice-used by Chinese to treat TB -dr. Kloss- drink 1 qt. Slippery elm tea daily -mix = part---comfrey, marshmallow, chickweed, and slippery elm–put 4 oz. Mixture to 4 qt. Water boil to 2 qt.- strain take ½ cup every 2 hours- hot/ cold

-*Swedish bitters*-take 1 tbs. Every morning for 6 weeks—noni

-Echinacea and goldenseal use mullein and red clover for cough and as an anti-tubercular antibiotic. Take one tablespoon each of Echinacea and goldenseal and boil gently for 25 minutes in one quart of water. Pour it all into a bowl containing one to two tablespoons each of red clover and mullein. Cover and steep for 30 minutes. Make fresh daily. One quart is one day's dosage.

TUMORS

Barley green helps to cure (black salve pulls tumors out)

Poultice -slice and heat figs (enough according to size of tumor) -make into paste (use enough castor oil to moisten figs) -apply very warm for 3 days .after 3 days over: (next 3 days)

-poke root (fresh)- wash and grind -make a flax seed /slippery elm tea enough to hold poke root together -add 3-4 tbsp. Blood root - apply over wound very warm(not hot) -leave on wound for 3 days (if bandage get soiled, change it, leaving on the plaster as much as possible)-next 3 days: -apply the fig /castor oil mixture-next 3 days: -alternate poke root mixture

Keep alternating every 3 days (tumor should start dropping off) (use cayenne or alum and goldenseal powders to stop bleeding and promote healing)

-sanicle* internal and external

Poultice-for external tumors -slippery elm/ sage

Herbs: plantain, chamomile, redroot, sassafras, chickweed, kelpgoldenseal, elder blossom, oregano, comfrey, mugwort, white oak dock root, flax seed, lobeliablue violet, skunk cabbage, skullcap, mullein, wild yam, red clover, hops, juniper berries, sageburdock, Echinacea bayberry, slippery elm

Vaginal: -slippery elm bark douche

Poultice: slippery elm, sage

Supplement: take vitamin-c to bowel tolerance

Supplements: -vitamin-e 1200 iu. Daily; -vitamin-c 1000mg daily; -kelp 5 tab 2x daily -niacin 50- 100 mg daily; -sarsaparilla tea - 1 tsp per cup 4x daily / 5 cap 3x daily; -poke root (break up hard calcified matter 1 cup of poke root to two qt. Water- boil for 5-10 minutes--take 1 cup 3x daily *chaparral

Cleanse – fast

Enema for 2 weeks before breakfast- or at bed time

Herbal formula: -St. John's wort -1 part; -chaparral -1 part; -alfalfa -2 parts; -pau d'arco -2 part;- violet leave -1 part -;Echinacea -2 part ;-kelp -1/3 part

Herbal formula: 6 1/2 cups of burdock root, 1 cup sheep sorrel, 1 oz. Turkey rhubarb root, 4 oz. Slippery elm

-mix dry ingredients together

-heat 2 oz. (4 tbsp.)-distilled water then mix it with 2 oz. Esiac tea mix below-

- bring 2 gallons of distilled to a boil in a stainlesskettle-allow brisk boil for 30 minutes

-put the mix into boiling water -stir and boil hard x 10 minutes

- allow to sit and cool slowly for 6 hours

-after 6 hours

-stir it thoroughly with a wooden or stainless tool

-let it sit for another 6 hours

-return the kettle to the stove and bring to a boil

-at the boiling point, turn heat off and strain into another kettle

-clean the kettle and pour content back in 1st pot-

-bottle while hot into dark glass and refrigerate

ULCER -Cheek and lip-check niacin deficiency	
ULCER (PEPTIC)	

Tea-flaxseed tea- 1tsp. In 1 cup boil h20 steep till gelatinous- drink at night

Formula ulcers: 1p each-slippery elm, marsh-mallow root, comfrey, goldenseal + ½ p lico-rice- place in #00 cap. Take 3 cap. 3x daily, after meal and before bed- on empty stomach (take comfrey 2-3 every hour during inflammation and burning then reduce to 2 every 4 hours

Dosages: It should be taken with hops or chamo-mile tea.

Cure takes three teaspoons of cayenne pepper per day. This cayenne may be mixed in water or tomato juice. It is recommended that you start with only 1/8 teaspoon three times a day, and then gradually work up to the one teaspoon three times a day.

Clay-1tbs in 6 oz. Water 3x daily + apply clay poultice 3x daily; silver biotic, sarsaparilla- cures

Aloe Vera -ulcers: use as part of treatment only. Take 2-4 t juice or gel 1/2 hour before meal time and before bedtime. -continue for 18 months-take 2-21/2 fluid dram doses or 1 tbsp. Every bedtime for 18 months

Diet-gastric ulcer: pumpkin, rice, avocado, ba-nana, okra, peach.

Acid self-test:-at pain-- take 1 tbsp. Lemon juice--if pain leaves= too little acid

-If symptoms worsen = too much acid---if you crave for sour foods, grape fruit=under acid

Ulcer pain:-ice bag above navel-2 cap cayenne pepper 2x daily, 1/3 cup aloe gel

-1 tbs. Slippery elm in small glass of water -golden seal and myrrh 1 tsp. Each 2x daily*For rapid pain relief,* drink a large glass of water. It dilutes the stomach acids and flushes them out.

Ulcer attack:-1/2 +1/2 potatoes juice and cab-bage juice give immediate relief

Cabbage: also several leafy green vegetables (has vitamin- u) -may mix 50-50 with carrot and / celery juice- drink ½ glass several times daily-cabbage juice 1 pt.1-2 times daily

-do not boil use the natural juice - vitamin-u is anti- ulcer-some people develop gas and bloat-ing but after the 5th day of treatment symptoms are rare-make the cabbage juice fresh (can last for 3 weeks when frozen) -take four to five 6-8 ounce servings

Diet: - eat several small meals -white rice and millet -6-8 olives with each meals

(avoid those canned in vinegar) -dried sweet al-monds - ripe olives:-4-6 with each meal -bland diet -doctors in India use dried bananas or fresh bananas -juice cabbage +celery +carrot juice will gives immediate relief

Herbs: sarsaparilla, marshmallow, licorice, slip-pery elm, chamomile, DGL, St. John's wort, mal-va, bilberry, flax, catnip, goldenseal ,bayberry, myrrh, aloe Vera, hops, skullcap, valerian-helps with sleep, yellow sweet clove

-strong tea from dried comfrey roots+ leaves take several times a day in an empty stomach

Hydrotherapy-skin ulcers -see local alternate bath-apply ice bag to the abdomen just

Above the navel or to the portion of the spine between the shoulder blades

-avoid cold spray -hot fomentation over stomach each night as needed

-hotsitz bath for pain as needed -heating trunk pack- for these conditions 20-25 minutes is the usual treatment time.

Supplement: vitamin-c -1000mg every 1 hour for 2 days (very healing) vitamin-a 25,000 iu. 2x daily, vitamin-e 600-1200 iu. 2x daily, brewer's yeast 2-3 tbs. 2xd ail ,zinc -15mg

Stomach ulcers:-1lb. Clay in 6 oz. Water 3x daily and apply to stomach 3x daily -cayenne pepper-yellow root-root tea-cabbage juice 1 pt.-white potatoes juice ½ pint -goldenseal 1 tsp. 2x daily-mix 1 glass of aloe gel with 1 glass of honey mix an equal amount of pure olive oil and put in a bottle- boil the bottle slowly for 3 hours- take 1 tbs. In the morning and 1 tbs. Before eating- keep cool **Leg ulcer:** apply clay poultice to area 3x daily **Baked potatoes** a mixture of 75% cabbage juice and 25% tomatoes juice-- raw potatoes juice drink emediately-6 oz. 2x daily	Vitamin-b complex including b12 300mg daily, chlorophyll tab. 3-5 tab 3x daily Cayenne 1-3 cap daily, vitamin-u-anti ulcer vitamin (cabbage) **Vomiting** -ice pills, distilled water **Ulceration suppository**: melt cocoa butter ads 2 tbs. White oak bark, 2 tbs. Acidophilus, 1 tsp each whey, myrrh- roll 2 / more suppositories in wax paper, refrigerate insert for at least 5 nights

ULCERS LEG

Flaxseed and charcoal may be used on sloughing ulcers or wounds. Use three tablespoons of powdered charcoal, three tablespoons or ground flaxseed and one cup of water. Thicken by bringing almost to a boil while stirring and apply in the usual way. **Clay poultice** -make 1 gallon very strong goldenseal tea – strain put leg in x 1 hour then let it air dry x10 minutes then apply olive oil in and around the ulcer then dust goldenseal powder on it-carrot poultice -flowering dogwood- use the root bark as poultice -sage wash and hot sage compress	**Make a gallon of goldenseal tea** (stronger than you would drink); and, after straining out the herb, put the leg in it for an hour. When finished, let it dry for 10 minutes; apply olive oil in, and around, the ulcer. Dust a little powdered goldenseal on it. If needed to keep out insects, put a light gauze bandage over it while letting the air in. It will heal, but slowly. As much as two months may be required. **Take garlic, vitamin -c** (1000mg) and vitamin-k (140mcg) multivitamin supplements

ULCERATIVE COLITIS

Ulcer of colon and liver-mix together the following and take 4 capsules 4x daily -cayenne 1 part -Echinacea 3 part-yellow dock 2 part -red clover 3 part -blue vervain 2 part -milk thistle 2 part -black cohosh 1 part -saffron 1 part -blue cohosh 2 part -comfrey 3 part -slippery elm 3 part -dandelion 3 part **Cabbage juice** -8 oz. Before meals **Bleeding-** hot enema (115-122 degrees far.) **Diarrhea**-carrots / carob/ banana -cooked brown rice water- **Enema daily**- 1tbs acidophilus in 10 oz. Water +/ golden seal enema-garlic enema(10 oz. Daily)	**Hydrotherapy:** fomentations to the abdomen once a day for 20 minutes with a hot foot bath. A hot retention enema given at about 109 to 110 degrees of goldenseal tea and pectin mixed. A cold sitz bath for 15-30 minutes with a hot foot bath may decrease diarrhea. *Hot bath nightly* -with (3 cups apple cider vinegar + 2 tbsp. Acidophilus for 3o minutes add 3tbs ginger to water *Cold sitz bath* 15-30 minutes- (92- 94 degrees f.)-with hot foot bath (108-122 degrees f **Inflammation** - charcoal compress made with strong hops tea instead of water. Applied at bedtime and left on all night. Drinking

Formula-*slippery elm* 4 cap daily / 1 tbsp. Powder 3x daily + chia seed 1 tbsp. 2x daily -*1 pint boiling water* + 1 tsp goldenseal +1/4 tsp myrrh take 1 tbsp. 6-8x daily **Teas:** peppermint, goldenseal, slippery elm,-- aloe Vera (1/2 cups daily) catnip, **Pain-** hot compress to abdomen, **suppository:-** melt coconut oil+ 2tbs of white oak bark + 1tbs whey +1 tsp myrrh(insert x 5 nights) **Diet:** no sugar + no oil-slippery elm tea, one teaspoon in one cup of very warm water. Take one cup three times a day at usual mealtimes even if skipping the meal.	-one tablespoon of crude pectin (canning variety) in a cup of water and stir it. Take three doses per day. -two goldenseal capsules three times a day. -two enteric coated peppermint oil capsules as needed for abdominal cramping. -one half teaspoon of licorice powder to one cup of water per day -charcoal, one tablespoon of powder stirred in water, with each loose stool. Take at least an hour before or after meals -aloe Vera, one - two ounces once or twice daily just before meals. -charcoal slurry water, three to four glasses a day is often very helpful. -cold compress for one to five minutes by simply wringing a large towel from ice water.

URINATIONS

-<u>do not</u> use juniper **Male urinary tract-** Take two or more morning and night, with parsley tea when possible. Cayenne-ginger-golden seal root-gravel root or queen of the meadow root, juniper berries-marshmallow root-parsley root or herb-uvaursi leaves-Siberian ginseng root **Albumin in the urine**: hot blanket pack/ other sweating treatments-repeat every 2-4 hours Hot Blanket Pack and other sweating measures to maintain cutaneous activity, repeated every 2-4 hours **Cystitis/ urinary tract infection:-** use of aluminum is a cause- symptom-lower back pain, frequent, urgent urination, urine strong and with unpleasant odor, appears cloudy (pus), desire to urinate even after bladder is emptied Check for kidney stones -pain- hot sitz- 2x daily x 20 minutes- to one of them add 1 cups of vinegar- to the next add juice of crushed strained garlic (2 cloves) -hot water bottle in direct contact with ureter, vaginal opening or heat lamp	**Scalding urine**: -cleanse-= parts fennel, burdock, slippery elm- steep 1 tsp x 20 minutes in 1 cup boiling water-drink 1 cold cupful with each meal and at night -tea of *cubeb berries is also excellent -*fleabane -yellow sweet clover **Pumpkin seed oil-** promotes healthy bladder *buchu **Entire urinary tract problem**: false unicorn* horsetail **Urine too acid**: -free use of fruit and water drinking in the forenoon .children cannot urinate: blend watermelon seeds and make tea give small amounts frequently ***Poor urine flow:***Take a cold sitz bath (cold partial bath, as you sit in the bathtub). Stop using salt. Drink 2 quarts a day of 50-50 orange juice and water - Corn-silk tea is the best; others include juniper berries, carrot tops, comfrey, plantain, cleavers, and chickweed. -Insert a soft catheter and draw out the urine.

-herbs; lovage, parsley, uvaursi, rupturewort, bearberry, birch, prickly ash, couch grass -horsetail-drink tea from 2-3 crushed garlic or blended bulbs several times daily. Avoid zinc and iron supplements until this problem is over

Diuretic herbs:-corn silk tea, celery seed, eat crushed parsley, agrimony, asparagus, balm of Gilead, barberry, bayberry, bistort, black cohosh, blue cohosh, bugleweed, kava kava, mullein, juniper berry, saw palmetto, valerian, white oak-eat grapes freely-dries juniper berries-raw onions to food

-formula-to improve excretion of urine = part fennel root, celery root, parsley root, asparagus root...steep 1 tsp in 1/2 cup boiling water, take 1/2-1 cup daily in mouthful doses

-formula---1/2tsp juniper berries, dandelion root, broom tops to a pint water-boil in low flame till it as down to 1/2 pint- strain put in jar-2 tbsp. 3x daily

Incontinence:-percussion douche to spine-neutral sitz bath x 15- 30 minutes-do exercise of sphincter muscle by stopping and releasing urine flow 1-2 seconds repeating 6-8 times as you urinate-double voiding is helpful- half way through stop and stand and sit and continue voiding leaning slightly at the knees

-herbs-when the disorder is not caused by (kidney stones, palsy, gout etc.) do this: mix = parts white oak bark, bistort root, valerian, sumac berries, white pond lily- steep 1 heaping tsp. In a cup of boiling water- drink 1 cup 1 hour before each meal and before retiring (4 cups a day) or take plantain tea for similar effect- increase dose if necessary

Incontinence: Percussion Douche to spine, Neutral Sitz Bath, 15-30 minutes

Nocturia: - *Revulsive*Sitz Bath. Begin at 100° and increase rapidly to 106°-115° F. (with a footbath at 110°-112° F.) For 3-8 minutes. Keep the head cool with cold cloths over forehead or around back of neck. Finish with a cold (55°-65° F.) Pail pour to hips

-Steep the following in a quart of boiling water: 1 tsp. Goldenseal and a half tsp. Each of boric acid and myrrh. Strain through a fine cloth, and inject through a fountain syringe. Retain as long as possible. You can moisten the tip with slippery elm tea.

-A cold shower often helps.

Stopped urine flow: Put the person to bed; give very warm high enema of catnip tea.

-apply hot fomentations, wrung out of smart-weed tea, to the bladder and lumbar region (small of back).

-Give 2-3 hot sitz baths in a bathtub, each day.

-An especially helpful remedy is a strong, hot as can be taken, tea of catnip, given as an enema. Drink it freely.

-hydrotherapy: hot blanket pack, dry sweating pack, cold/ hot sitz bath for 5 minutes, cold shower often help, cold perennial douche, cold douche to lower back, front and back, opposite the intestines and pelvic organs, cold rubbing sitz bath

-use no salt-drink 2 qt. 50-50 orange juice and water-if bed ridden--short cold water over perennial, genitals, and entire length of spine

-herbs: corn silk, carrot tops, cleavers, juniper berries, comfrey, plantain, chickweed -high enema of catnip tea -steep- 1 tsp goldenseal + 1/2 tsp each boric acid and myrrh-strain, and inject in rectum with syringe

Cold shower helps-steep 1 heaping tsp yarrow in a cup boiling water x 20 min. Drink 1 cup cold before each meal10-insert a catheter and let urine flow out

Horsetail grass 1/3 cup + elderberries 1/3 cup mix with 1 pt. Of water-make tea take 4 oz. 3x daily

Difficulty passing urine- Tea-1 oz. Couch grass+ 1 oz. Buchu+ 1 oz. Marshmallow in 1 ½ pt. H20 simmer for 15 min. -1 cup 4 times daily

Cant urinate-rub the loins with onion to increase elimination by 25%

UTERUS

See fibroid section

Herbal-a=acute; sa=subacute; c=chronic; d=degenerative

A-(itching, burning, rash) goldenseal, myrrh, yarrow, comfrey, garlic

Sa-(menstrual problems) blue cohosh, uvaursi, burdock, dong quai, goldenseal, chaparral, cohosh

C-(cyst) Echinacea, burdock, cayenne, uvasanicle

D-(degenerative stage , VD) cayenne, goldenseal, chaparral, uvaursi

Uterine bleeding

Hot vaginal irrigation; short Hot Hip Pack; Hot Footbath, followed by Cold Compress over stomach and inner surfaces of thighs. In obstinate cases, cold vaginal irrigation. Moderately prolonged, very cold, Shallow Sitz Bath at 50^0-65^0 F. For 5-15 minutes, accompanied by Hot Footbath when other measures fail; hot Douche to lower spine area over stomach and inner surfaces of thighs, twice daily during intervals.

__Caution__: Cold applications must not be used in cases excessive bleeding during menstruation

VAGINAL

Herbal-a=acute; sa=subacute; c=chronic; d=degenerative

A-(itching, burning, rash) goldenseal, myrrh

Sa(yeast infestation, leucorrhea, fungus) goldenseal, burdock, onion, geranium, blue violet, myrrh

D-(degenerative stage, Venereal Disease) uvaursi, burdock, Mormon tea, chaparral, goldenseal

Vaginal YEAST

Herbs include pau d'arco tea as a natural antibiotic. Drink 3 cups daily.

Yeast infection, or vaginal infection, take three cups apple cider vinegar, put it in a tub of water. Bring the water up around the hips. Have the sister sit in the tub with her legs flexed. The apple cider vinegar will actually discourage and destroy the pathogenic bacteria, and the yeast bacteria

-**Beware of tub baths!** Take showers instead.

-Tea tree oil is good for vaginitis. Use creams, suppositories, etc.

-Aloe Vera is helpful for infections, including yeast infections. It can be taken internally or used as a douche. -Also helpful are bayberry, goldenseal, yarrow, marshmallow root, calendula, chamomile, pau d'arco, and dandelion.

-To normalize vaginal flora, eat plain yogurt and/ or apply it to the vagina.

If you have chronic or persistent vaginitis, you may have diabetes.

-If you have recurring vaginitis, you may be getting it from your husband

Vaginal infection:-week before nightly- day- 1 insert garlic clove in vagina at night

Day-2 bruise garlic then insert

Day-3 cut dents in garlic with knife then insertdo this 6 nights- skip 1 day then start--suppository- goldenseal, yellow dock, poke root 2t+ 1t slippery elm and garlic- put 4-6 dropper full of t-tree oil (not drops) into herbs-+ pinch cayenne add coconut oil(liquid) to make dry pie dough— make 12 large suppositories(freeze)—administer nightly for 6 nights—in am douche with 1 oz. Lemon juice per qt. Water—stop 1 day and repeat cycle 3x of garlic and suppository for severe infections

-*For yeast vaginitis,* use a hot soda-water douche (1-3 teaspoons of soda to 1 quart water) twice a day for 7 days, then once a day for 30 days.
• If there is not clear and rapid improvement, a *trichomonas may be the* cause. If so, apply a vinegar douche (1-4 tablespoon of vinegar to 1 quart water) twice a day for 7 days, then once a day for 30 days.

-Garlic-water douche (1 clove into part of a quart of boiling water; add the remainder of the quart, let cool to 110° F. Twice a day for 7 days, then once a day for 30 days). • For organisms other than yeast and trichomonas, a warm normal saline douche (1 teaspoon of salt per quart water) is useful.

-Hot sitz baths, 2-3 times a day will soothe local irritation; but it is important that the tub be sterilized first, lest bacteria be introduced into the vagina.

-Take vitamins A and B complex.

WARTS -cause=virus	
Skin, vocal cords, genital-4-6 ounces of savoy cabbage juice daily. If you can find indole-3-carbinol in a health food store, add a teaspoon to any kind of juice two to three times daily instead of the cabbage juice.	**Apply powdered vitamin-c**, as paste and cover take vitamin-e and put it on area- .
	Clove oil
Water proof adhesive x 6 1/2 days, scratch it and repeat each time	**Take supplements**: vitamin-a, e b- complex, zinc
Poultice:-herbs: comfrey, milkweed, celandine, green fig leaves, marigold, corn cockle	**Diet:** lots of garlic and onions
	Warts plantar -vitamin-e oil apply nightly, use 500mg vitamin-c in water and make paste (may take 2 months), use garlic with warm castor oil in gauze- apply 3x daily, use dandelion milk/ milkweed 3x daily, fig milk will remove wart fast-drops of castor oil-a hot foot bath
Onion set in the apple cider vinegar at least five or six hours and then you take it out. You simply apply that over the wart and wrap it.	
Sour apple juice:+few grain Epson salt and follow adhesive procedure on	**Warts venereal** -drink- 2 cups of pau d'arco and Echinacea tea daily-take daily calcium supplement to prevent it from turning cancerous-take 10 drops of grape seed extract daily
White cabbage juice / aloe pulp/ garlic/ raw potatoes/ 2x daily x several weeks	
Banana skin : -daily for 6 weeks-	-Bathe sores several x daily with goldenseal myrrh solution
Castor oil: (works better when old and rancid)-2x daily x 3 weeks-k-cover area with	-Vaginal suppository- of t-tree oil nightly or use goldenseal/ chaparral suppository mixed with vitamin-a-alt. Hot cold fomentation, baths, sitz to pelvic area
Garlic:- tape a piece to area -2 tbs. + 1 tbs. Warm castor oil- apply 3x daily--m-muriatic acid: - 1 drop 2x daily x 3 weeks-- n-garlic and warm castor oil:-on gauze 3x daily	
	Plantar warts (warts on the bottom of your foot), apply a plantain poultice (the leaf itself) to the wart
Green fig milk(barely ripe):will remove warts fast-	
WOUND	
Immediately- take vitamin-c 5000mg, .apply-t-tree oil to prevent infection (every 3 hours)	**Application:** calendula*comfrey root, Echinacea, plantain, goldenseal, soak bandage with aloe Vera ---result no scar
Accident wound / injury- boil the grapefruit for five to ten minutes in water with Epsom Salt (3 cups to one grapefruit); take out the meat of the grapefruit. Put a little Epsom Salt on. Marinate grapefruit in the Epsom Salt. The grapefruit is covered with Epsom Salt. Open wounds, broken bones that have been reset but still have a lot of pain, any type of severe pain and especially open wounds. Take the grapefruit and put it on the kneecap and bandage it. If you apply it quickly after using ice you will not need stitches. Use Crazy Glue to close clean	**Bleeding-***sprinkle alum- will stop bleeding. Immediately*
	Fenugreek poultice*.horehound- poultice, wrap papaya leaves, or wheat grass on area, yellow sweet clover
	Inflammation or redness- apply goldenseal
	Diabetic wound: powdered goldenseal , sugar to wound, vit-e 1000 daily/ hot and cold bath
	Sugar poultice-Use for infection ulcers- disinfects- Pour in gangrene/ cancer wound- it will melt keep pouring until stops- then clean area and apply goldenseal latter on put myrrh to form scab
Comfrey compress.	

Flaxseed and charcoal may be used on sloughing ulcers or wounds. Use three tablespoons of powdered charcoal, three tablespoons or ground flaxseed and one cup of water. Thicken by bringing almost to a boil while stirring and apply in the usual way.

-**clay, noni. Zinc**- promote healing, infected with fever- see blood poisoning apply cayenne

Hydrotherapy: - infected wound add peroxide to water (see local alternate bath)

Slow healing-- barley green* -zinc supplements -take Swedish bitters -need vitamin-f (flaxseed)

Antiseptic- grapefruit

Topical

Gangrene severe- hot and cold until it bleeds than apply sugar treatment

Pour in gangrene/ cancer wound- it will melt keep pouring until stops- then clean area and apply goldenseal latter on put myrrh to form scab

Gangrene severe- hot and cold until it bleeds than apply sugar treatment

Crazy glue- for suture Wound/ accident/ injured bone 1st apply ice when severe bleed stop with pressure apply

Grapefruit poultice

1st pull it out of the skin without destroying the skin

Boil grapefruit in water and 3 cups of Epson salt, remove from pot and marinate or cover with Epson salt - you will put it back in the skin

PART THREE
DIETETIC PRINCIPLES

Meals-regularity in meals: maintain a regular schedule-do not eat too early or too late

-with severe illness- go on a total raw diet for months

Moderation:-only as much as you need -never overeat-only eat to satisfy hunger and then stop

Eat-take small bites:-only put a small amount in your mouth at a time-you will chew and salivate it better-you will tend to eat less in a meal-relax and *eat slowly*:-if you are too rush to eat , then don't eat-do not be worried, anxious, fatigued, hurried or angry-

*Chew*your food well:-you will derive more energy out of less food if you do this-

Do not eat too many things at one meal:-three or four items is sufficient

Avoid complicated mixtures:-say no to the gravies, vegetable loaves, gluten foods, keep your meal simple

Avoid peculiar additives:-vinegar, monosodium glutamate, etc.(they upset the stomach and slow digestion)

Vary your diet from meal to meal: if you ate oatmeal in the morning try rye tomorrow

The food should be palatable:-if it is good food this should not be difficult

Never eat food prepared in aluminum:-or drink water from aluminum containers

(Alzheimer's is worth avoiding)

Drink all water between meals:-not with meals-except for fresh fruit / vegetable juice

As a rule:-eat fruits and vegetables in separate meals-except for citrus can be eaten with either

Greens have more compacted vitamin. And minerals than other type of foods:

Fresh fruits (not cooked) -eat raw-do not eat melons, cantaloupes, watermelons with other meals

-always soak dried fruits before eating (prunes, apricots etc.).-never eat sulfured food

Grains:-only eat whole, unprocessed grains-avoid processed grain White flour)

-if you eat wheat (make zwieback)- toast until firm but not rock hard (more digestible)

-avoid toasted wheat germ (oils will be rancid) (raw wheat germ should be stored in refrigerator)

-oats are the best grain (eat rye, millet, buck-wheat) Cheerios -eat unpolished brown rice

Nuts and seeds:-eat fresh-chew very well-eat sparingly (handful daily)

-avoid peanut butter with hydrogenated vegetable oils

Fats:-best flax oil (for vitamin -F)- barlean brand-sunflower seed oil, soy oil, corn oil are second best -wheat germ oil -never eat cotton seed oil

Sweetener:-use fresh fruits - little honey or black-strap molasses-sweet tooth - take a little molasses after meals

Other nutrients: -salt- use sparingly or not at all (best to add salt after food is cooked)

(only iodized salt)- use dulse or kelp -nova scotia dulse- full of trace minerals use to replace salt (Norwegian kelp is an alternate-use herbs for seasoning

-cayenne-too much can lead to pleurisy

Vegetables: -best raw -green drinks good-steam for little time only

-use vegetable water for broth or soups-do not peel potatoes, beets, squash

-they only lack vitamin-D (you get this from sunlight) -but they don't have adequate trace minerals **Nova scotia dulse and Norwegian kelp** :-(are 2 types of seaweed) are the only rich source of trace minerals **Blackstrap molasses**:-is the only very rich source of iron -it is very rich in choline and inositol, (the 2 B-vitamins used in large quantities **Best pattern:-**rest before the meal-and walk around after it not vice versa	-avoid too much spinach (oxalic acid)-never eat rhubarb (high in oxalic acid)-fiber important (oat bran best)

PART FOUR
AT ONSET OF ILLNESS

Catnip-make a strong tea of catnip- soak a hand towel in the tea wring it out and place over the lower abdomen-**sea salt-** 2 tsp. To 1 qt. Of pure warm water- drink all

Cleanse-All diseases- (parasite, liver, kidney, blood, colon cleanse to avoid relapse of disease)

Cure-most disease are curedwith fasting, simple diet, rest and water therapy , enemas (herbs a last resort)

Diet-change to a 75-100% raw diet 100% raw if severe illness such as Cancer)

Eight laws-obey the **8 laws** of health

Fast for 3+ days -At symptoms of any disease, while doing a cleanse-at least 3 days fasting will lead to great results fasting(juice/ water/ simple foods)

Healing process must be gradual transition back to regular living-trying to make the system too pure too fast can overly weaken the person

Shrubs-No shrubs close to house, or numerous shade trees-avoid water running close to dwelling place

Sick room should be well ventilated (no draft)

Stove heat-destroys the vitality of the air and weakens the lungs -heat oppressed atmosphere, deprives vitality and benumbs brains, lungs, liver

Supplements-clay- Swedish bitters- used to treat a variety of different diseases

Esiac tea- for *cancer*

Mineral and vitamin supplement- study shows some diseases are a result of deficiency- due to depleted soils and poor diet

D. Noni- this plant has been used to treat a variety of different diseases

E. Nutritional deficiency-all diseases has its foundation in some sort to deficiency

- if you are not eating food from good soil- you are depleted - start taking vitamins from whole food concentrate or barley green (superfood)

PART FIVE
TOXIC ITEMS

ADDITIVES OF FOOD: Leads to arthritis, cardiac, and cancer problems causes anemia

ALCOHOL, DRUGS: Causes-liver disease, cardiac disease-Depletes body from B- vitamins and some minerals

-causes bleeding from stomach -causes infertility by causing the female egg not to be implanted in uterus

ALUMINUN: Cooking or eating food in aluminum linked to Alzheimer's

ANTIDEPRESSANTS: (aluminum)- Alzheimer's

PERMANENT HAIR DYES (some linked to cancer)

CAFFEINE PRODUCTS: see meat, coffee, cheese -increases cortisol level causes increase aging process

-decreases iron in the blood 70% -makes it more difficult for the body to absorb iron-blocks calcium absorption

BAKING POWDER AND SODA: damage the lining of the stomach

BIRTH CONTROL PILLS: -causes phlebitis

BRA (wearing more than 12 hours daily-specially wire bras)

BREAST IMPLANTS- linked to breast cancer

CHEESE: Process is very unhealthy use a little yogurt to normalize stomach flora

CHLORINATED WATER: El.DRINKING/ POOL

Leads to atherosclerosis, can cause colon cancer, cause hyperactivity in children

CADMIUM - found in city water linked to high blood pressure (large amount found in kidneys of those that die from

High blood pressure blocks entrance of iodine in the thyroid

CHOCOLATE- contains oxalic acid and prevents the absorption of calcium

MERCURY (AMALGAN FILLINGS, FISH) -inhibit DNA repair, alters cells ability to receive nutrient/ exchange material hinder function enzymes, produce non

-functional chemicals, interferes with nerve impulses, interferes endocrine function, kill digestive bacteria,

-symptoms- tremors, depression, fatigue, irritability, moodiness, nervous excitability, loss of memory, inability to concentrate, insomnia, drowsiness, loss of appetite, birth defects, miscarriages, nephritis, kidney disease, pneumonitis, ulceration of oral mucosa, swollen glands and tongue, loosening of teeth, dark pigmentation of gums

-treatment-remove them 1-800-leadout (biologist dentist)- to find a doctor near you, take nutritional supplements for a

Few months prior to removal, take heavy metal detox for 6 months after (cholera, garlic, vitamins, minerals, amino acids, vitamin-c, MSM, milk thistle, DMSA, sauna hydrotherapy treatments)

MILK AND MEAT: contaminated and disease-fish- diseased and high mercury lever -meat has a high phosphorus content which leads to calcium deficiency (phosphorus binds with calcium) -high protein diet causes calcium loss

MONO AND DICICLERIDE= pork products

MOUTHWASH: -25% alcohol -causes cancer

MSG: -cytotoxic, with glutamic acid- which allows increase calcium in brain and eats holes in brain, similar to what nutrasweet does to the system-causes reproductive, birth defect problems

-proven to cause permanent brain damage in children (removed from baby food)

NICOTEINE PRODUCTS:-cancer and other hazards produced -causes phlebitis-destroys vitamin -c in the body

COD LIVER OIL: it contains too much vitamin A and D

-cosmetics / shaving cream etc. By law manufacturers are allowed to place 25 % hidden (non-labeled toxic ingredients in

Your cosmetics

-with 100's of chemicals -propylene glycol -found in antifreeze -brake fluid -found in baby wipes

-causes dermatitis -kidney disease

-shaving cream- propane, butane -cosmetics- have 1/3 hidden- ingredients not on label

COW'S MILK/ MEAT-diseased, depletes the body from calcium, increase protein causes same

DECAFFEINATED COFFEE- linked to spontaneous abortion

FOOD- WORST FOOD ADDITIVES

-BHN (butylated hydroxyanisole) food preservative ,allergies, liver disease, cancer

-caffeine-coloring, flavoring, stimulant

-nervousness, heart palpitation and defect

-caramel-

-genetic defect, possible cancer

-carrageen-thickening agent, binder

-colitis, genetic defects

-EDTA Preservative, food coloring (calcium disodium ethylenediamine tetraacetate)

-kidney disorder, cramps, skin rash, intestinal problems

-gums: Arabic, thickener, binder, increase easy flow, cellulose, ghatti karaya, tragacanth, xanthan

-allergic reactions, constipation, diarrhea

-hydroxylated lecithin-binder

-skin irritations

-lactic acid-preservative

-caustic

-maltol dextrin- aroma and flavor enhancer

-derived from harmful wood tars

-modified food starch, thickener, filler

OXALC CID-HIGH OXALIC ACID FOODS (lead to bone loss)- pilchard, spinach, rhubarb, poke

ORAL CONTRACEPTIVES- (women that uses it have 3x higher chance for breast cancer)

PRESERVATIVES- are rich in phosphorus and locks with calcium and carries it out of the body

PORK ADDITIVES- lard

emulsifiers , animal shortening

stabilizers(mono+diglyserides)

gelatin, tween ,shortening

swine pepsin, animal fats

calcium stearate

hydrolyzed animal protein/ protein

Collagen or enzyme

magnesium stearate, tallow

poly-sorbates, monostearates

fatty acids

PROCESSED FOODS -include "food" found in the store

-are rich in phosphorus- locks with calcium and carries it out of the body (weak bones)

SALT- even if it states sea salt- make sure it does not contain aluminum (call the company)use nova scotia dulse

SHARK CARTILEDGE: may inhibit production of new blood cells needed to increase blood circulation

SHELLFISH:-20-30 people die per year with arsenic poisoning from shellfish

-fish has increased level of arsenic

SOAP: by law manufactures are allowed to put 25% hidden, non-labeled toxic ingredients in the soap

-has sodium loral sulfate- (makes soap foam) causes damaged skin-causes permanent eye damage

-canker sores -FDC blue eye #1 (carcinogenic)

SODA'S: = phosphoric acid - it locks up with calcium and makes it unavailable, causes

-vomiting, lung damage

-monoglycerides and diglycerides

-genetic changes, cancer birth defects

Softener, smoothing agents

-MSG(monosodium glutamate) flavoring enhancer

-headaches, chilling, sweating ,diarrhea, chest pain, genetic damage

-nitrites sodium nitrite, preservative, coloring, curing -cancer causing

-polysorbate 60, 65, 80 Emulsifier for creaminess

-diarrhea

-propyl gallate- preservative

-liver damage, birth defect

-propylane glycol alginate , thickener, stabilizer

-liver damage

-red dye-40 (allura red ac) coloring

-birth defect cancer

-saccharin-sugar substitute

 -allergic response, effect skin, heart, Intestine, tumors , bladder cancer

-sodium erythrobate- preservative, coloring agent -genetic defect

-tannin (tanic acid)-flavoring

-liver ailment, tumors, cancer

FLUORIDE (uses for rat poisoning) /chlorine:- thyroid gland absorbs them

-Why are the warning labels on toothpaste?- causes hyperactivity in children -causes low IQ in children

-carcinigenic, bone cancer, oral cancer, tumors, Arthritis, allergy-does not prevent cavities

-Europe have stopped chlorinated water be- cause of the disease risk (95% of the water is not chlorinated)
-injures bones teeth and nerves

GRAVIES: -pastries, ice cream, etc.

GUM CHEWING causes stomach acid to keep flowing - weakening the stomach, causes ulcers

Magnesium and calcium deficiency-is more acid than vinegar- it removes calcium and carries it off

-the high sugar content irritates the nerves -pulls calcium out of the bones

SODIUM NITRITES; -found in meat and is con- verted to methianine -causes Alzheimer's, cancer

SOFT DRINKS:-contains phosphoric acid which locks with calcium and carries it out of the body leading to Weak bones

-leaches calcium from bones- a tooth placed in a cola drink disappeared in a few hours

SPICES AND CONDIMENTS: (pepper, mustard, cinnamon, etc.)- linked to intestinal cancer

SUGAR: clogged the system, Debilitating, do not use white sugar, Contributes to endometriosis

SUGAR -ARTIFICIAL: CAUSES BRAIN LEISIONS-nutrasweet:(aspartame)

-concerts to methal alcohol- found in paint thin- ner -found in diet soda

-causes seizures, brain tumors - (diet soda) +so- dium nitrite(meat) :

-forms DPK- which breaks to nitro-urea-which causes malignant brain tumors in lab animals

-cyclamate: found in artificial sugar- causes blad- der tumor -causes anemia

-decreases immune system by 50%

TALC: -ovarian cancer- (found in infant powder) -lung irritation -asbestos

VINEGAR: is a powerful acid -destroys stomach

VITAMIN-D SUPPLEMENT: can cause colon cancer

VEGETABLE (RHUBARB)- do not eat it is too high in oxalic acid- spinach ,don't eat too much - oxalic acid blocks calcium absorption in the body

WHITE FLOUR PRODUCTS: (cookies, dough- nuts, soda crackers, biscuits, bread, bagels)

-forms a glue and is hard on the digestive tract -contributes to endometriosis

HYDROGENATED OILS: (AVOID GREESE, FRIED FOODS) -causes cancer, increase cholesterol, decrease sperm count, breast cancer -coats the arteries and produces fat cells -avoid fried foods-changes the oil to trans-fat (causes heart disease) -they produce fat cells **IRON SUPPLEMENTS**- accelerate cancer growth **INSECTICIDES:-**destroy bone marrow- causing no new red blood cells **JUNK FOOD:** -debilitates the entire system -no nutrition-obesity -disease forming chemicals **MEAT:** -Carries diseases-are rich in phosphorus which locks with calcium carrying it out of the body leading to weak bones **MEDICATIONS**:-seek alternatives-destroys vitamins(especially-e vitamin) and minerals in the body	**YEAST -BAKERS YEAST**: except brewer's or torula yeast

PART SIX
ACID- ALKALI FOODS

ALKALINE FOODS 70%	ACID FOODS 30%
Alfalfa	Alcohol
Almonds	Barley
Apples	Beef, all kinds
Apricots	Bread, all
Artichokes	Buckwheat
Asparagus	Candy
Avocados	Cheese, all
Bamboo shoots	Cherries
Bananas	Chicken
Beans, dried, green, lima	Codfish
Beans, soy	Corn, canned
Beans, string	Cornmeal
Beets, fresh	Coffee
Beet greens	Crackers
Berries, all	Cranberries
Brazil nuts	Eggs
Brocoli	Fowl
Cabage	Frog legs
Cantaloup	Gelatin
Carrots	Goose
Carob	Haddock
Cauliflower	Halibut
Celery	Ham
Chard	Hominy
Cherry juice	Jams and jellies
Citron	Flavorings
Coconuts	Lentils
Collards	Liver
Cucumbers	Lobster
Currants	Macaroni
Dandelion	Mayonnaise
Dates	Oatmeal

Eggplant	Oysters
Endive	Peanuts
Figs	Plums
Garbanzos	Prunes
Garlic	Rice
Grapes	Salmon
Grape juice	Shrimp
Grapefruit	Tapioca
Guava	Turkey
Honey	Veal
Honeydew	Vinegar
Kale	Walnuts
KohlrabiLeeks	Wheat
Légumes, exceptlentils	
Lettuce	
Mangoes	
Maple syrup	
Milk, soy	
Millet	
Melons, all	
Molasses	
Mushrooms	
Okra	
Olives	
Onions	
Oranges	
Orange juice	
Papayas	
Parsley	
Parsnips	
Peaches	
Peas, dried, fresh	
Pears	
Peppers, green	
Pineapple	
Potatoes, all	
Pumpkin	
Radishes	

Raisins

Rhubarb (oxalic acid)

Rutabagas

Sauerkraut:(lemon only)

Soybeans

Spinach

Squash

Strawberries

Tomatoes

Tomato juice

Tangerines

Turnips and tops

Watercress

Water chestnuts, fresh

PART SEVEN
GOD'S PLAN

GOD'S PLANS	EIGHT LAWS OF HEALTH
G- Golden SUNSHINE = 20-60 minutes daily	**N**- nutrition
O- Outdoor AIR = breathe deeply daily	**E**- exercise
D- Daily EXERCISE = progressive, walking, cycling, etc. At least 20 minutes 6x/ week	**W**- water
S- simple TRUST in god = daily devotions, study his word	**S**- sunshine
P - Plenty of REST = rise and retire at set times	**T**- temperance
L- Lots of WATER = 8 cups between meals (1/2 of your body's weight in ounces daily)	**A**-air
A- Always TEMPERATE = no junk foods, rich snacks, caffeine, nicotine, night life	**R**-rest
N - NUTRITIOUS foods = fruits, vegetables, grains, nuts (seeds largely) , 2-3 meals at set times , no nibbling ,	**T**- trust in Gd
S- SIMPLE dress = Keep extremities warm and covered	

PART EIGHT
FORMULA, TEA MAKING, TINCTURE

FORMULA Charcoal Teas Tinctures Rocket fuel Suppositories	

<table>
<tr><td>

HOW TO MAKE TEAS

Leaves Blossoms and-1 cup water+ 1 teaspoon Steep for

30 minutes

Powder1 cup water+½ teaspoon- Steep for 15 minutes

Bark, roots And seeds-1 cup water +1 tablespoon Boil gently for 20 minutes

Pau d'arco1 cup water +1 tablespoon -Boil gently for 10 minutes and steep for 20 minutes

EXTRACT- *use vinegar/ alcohol-you may use ordinary rubbing alcohol if for external use-*mix 1 ounce of herb with 1 pint of solution, shake once or twice a day for 2-3 weeks, strain and squeeze (if using alcohol mix with sufficient water to make 30% solution 60% proof alcohol is 30%

TINCTURES- 1-2 ounces of dried herbs steep in 1 pint of brandy/ vodka for 2 days- shake daily- then strain and store (use 1 tbs. 3 times daily)

ANTISPASMODIC TINCTURE

For seizures, cough etc.

-lobelia tincture 1 0z -skullcap tincture 1 oz. -skunk cabbage tincture (if available)-1 oz. -myrrh tincture 1 oz. -black cohosh tincture 1 oz. - cayenne pepper 1 tsp

-(mix give 8-15 drops in 1/2 glass water, if can't drink place under tongue)

</td><td>

CAYENNE PEPPER TINCTURE:

Note: parts equals volume

-Take a quart canning jar and fill it 1/4 full with dried cayenne peppers, 200,000+ heat units), that you can obtain.

-Add only enough 50% grain alcohol(100 proof vodka) to cover the cayenne peppers, which have been chopped fine, using a blender or grinder.

-Use enough fresh cayenne peppers, that you can blend with 50% grain alcohol (100 proof vodka) to turn the mixture into an apple sauce-like consistency.

Note: if you can't find 100 proof grain alcohol, then use 190 proof grain alcohol and dilute it by 50% with distilled water.

-Add this mixture to the 1st mixture, filling up the canning jar 3/4 full.

-Fill up the rest of the canning jar with more 50% grain alcohol.

-Shake it as many times as possible, during the day.

-Let this mixture sit, until the following full moon (15-16 days), but optimally until the following new moon (28-29 days)!

-Strain this mixture through an unbleached coffee filter.

-Bottle the resulting tincture.

-Take 2-3 dropperfuls - 3-4 times per day, when needed.

</td></tr>
</table>

CHARCOAL

Making charcoal:-the harder the wood the stronger and denser the charcoal-coconut shell makes excellent charcoal

Process:-heat at high temperature (80-1200 c) from 6-10 hoursin a furnace without oxygen

14 Capsules= 1 tbs.

Charcoal and smartweed-A handful of smartweed leaves in blender with ¼-1/2 cup water-chop coarsely- pour into a cup containing 1 tbs. Charcoal- mix and use as poultice

Charcoal and flaxseed/ psyllium = part

Charcoal and flax seed: 3 tbs. Grind milled flax + 1 tbs. Charcoal+ 1 cup water- mix and bring to a boil till thicken

Charcoal slurry- 1 tbs. Mixed in 4 cups water- allow to settle- drink clear top (good for infants and children also)

Charcoal castor oil fomentation:3 tbs. Charcoal+ 2 tbs. Flaxseed+ ½ tbs. Castor oil mix apply on cloth and heat up

Procedure for applying poultice- place on saran wrap and cover with saran and use a roll pin to make it at least ¼ inch thick (refrigerate for future use)- apply poultice on skin then wrap with saran then cloth

HERBAL SUPPOSITORIES

-Mix together the following ingredients: 1 heaping tablespoon. Of golden seal root (finely powdered), yellow dock (finely powdered), cayenne pepper powder, and freshly grated poke root, plus 6 droppersful (200 drops) - tea tree oil, & coconut oil (enough to make this mixture into pie-dough consistency).

-Form this mixture by rolling it back and forth between the palms of your hands, making 12 large or 24 medium suppositories.

-Place them on a glass plate into the freezer, until you need them.

ROCKET FUEL: blend together-1- medium onion +1-2 tbsp. Powdered ginger (or 1 1/2 piece) + 6-8 lemon +5 garlic cloves + pinch cayenne honey to taste +horse radish

PART NINE
CLEANSE

Do Three day cleanse then do mucus elimination diet- -every AM-drink 16 ounces or more of *prune juice* (unsweetened, if possible). -30 minutes later-and 8 oz. Of *distilled* water -repeat the juice and distilled water each 30 minutes throughout the day. -consume 1 gallon of apple juice each day - use prune juice of a colon cleanse during the 3-days -*take one or two tablespoons of olive oil three times a day* **-***On the fourth and subsequent days,* begin taking vegetable and fruit juices, along with raw fruits and vegetables.	**Mucus elimination diet** -*Do's:* Any whole, live, raw foods. Fruits, vegetables, whole grains, nuts, seeds, -*Don'ts*: Salt, eggs, all refined sugars, meat, all milk products, flours and flour products. **-***Breakfast- fresh fruit or a good low heated whole grain.* (With life in it). It can be prepared in a thermos bottle: Take a thermos bottle, fill in the early afternoon or evening one-third full of grain, and finish filling the thermos bottle with boiling water. Shake to mix the grain and water. The next morning the grain is ready for consumption. *Sprouted grains are excellent.* Use variety of grains. -*use Fruit and vegetable juices along with dried fruits,* use salads
Blood purify -½ oz. Elder, +1/2 oz. Peppermint in 1 pt. H20 -*Tea*-1 oz. Clover+1/2 oz. Burdock and ¼ oz. Sassafras in 1 qt. H20 poured hot over herbs-let stand for 1 hr. Take 1 cup 4 times daily -*Tea*-1 oz. Yellow dock+ ½ oz. Poke root+ ½ oz. Elder flower + 1 oz. Red clover in 1 qtr. Water-simmer x 15 min –I cup 4 times daily -Tea-1 oz. Burdock, 1 oz. Centaury+ ½ each yellow dock + bittersweet+ ¼ oz. Cayenne boil in 3 pt.- 1 cup 4 times daily h20 for 10 minutes *Acidosis*- yellow dock tea *Arthritis*-alfalfa seed tea *Eczema*; yellow dock tea *Enema*-flaxseed tea- 1 tbs. In 1 pt. Water boil 6-7 minutes *Fevers*- parsley seed tea *Gas*- pennyroyal and ginger tea for gas expel *Glands*- black cohosh tea-parsley and licorice tea	**REJUVELAC (PROBIOTIC)** *Loaded with vitamin B, K, E , protein and enzymes* Take 1 cup of wheat berries / other grain quinoa + rye makes the best Sprout just till tail starts-Let stand on counter for 24 hours rinsing it 3x during the 24 hours Place in large jar add 4 cups of water let stand for 2-3 days, strain and refrigerate Opt. Adds more water to grain it will make more in 24 hours. **YEAST OVERGROWTH & LEAKY GUT SYNDROME** *First procedure: On the first two days consume two quarts of a decoction of Black Walnut and Pau d' Arco (*one quart each day). This is made by simmering the herbs in water for twenty minutes at the rate of one tablespoon of the combined herbs (equal parts) per cup of water. This will kill off the yeast; can make you feel very nauseous. This nauseous feeling is avoided by taking plant-based *digestive enzymes* in large amounts (triple the stated dosages on the label) do enemas 1st two days

Mouth ulcers and throat-sorrel tea

Nerves- silicon, shave grass tea, oat straw tea

BOWEL-colon cleanse formula: 2cups alfalfa+ 2c psyllium husk + 1c slippery elm + 1c apple fiber + 1c Senna + 1/2 c charcoal + 1 tsp. Cayenne + 1/2 c wormwood/ 1/2 c black walnut mix- add bentonite clay 1/2 cup if taking colonics

Formula-mix psyllium 1 lb., slippery elm ½ lb., bran 1/3 lb.- take 1 tbs. In 6 oz. Of juice 3x daily

Pomegranate juice- 1 qt. Cleanses

Soak slices of cucumber in sea salt water- refrigerate drink 6 ounces before breakfast x3 days.

Soak prunes with 1 tbsp. Lemon juice + 1 tbsp. Honey + 1 tsp sea water - drink 4-5 ounces before breakfast

1/2 pounds of salt + 1 pounds chopped cabbage let stand x 1 hour- squeeze juice out drink 1/2 glass daily

Sea water 1 tsp in 6 oz. Of cabbage juice- drink in morning before breakfast

Chlorophyll- deodorizes the bowel damaged bowel tissue- it- helps build the tissues back

White oak bark- other cleansing enema option--white oak bark decoction nightly for 3 days

Sea salt water flush for 10 days with juicing for severe ill (2 ½ cups cold water+ 1 1/2 cups hot water + 1 tsp sea salt)- drink 2 of these within 15-20 minutes-Blend vegetables and drink without straining -Or sea salt water (2 level rounded tsp. Sea salt to 1 qt. Like warm water) drink within 30 minutes- first thing in the morning)- do not use iodized salt-10 day- cleanse-do not do sea salt cleanse if hypertensive, kidney disease, cancer, cardiac disease

CASTOR OIL PACK- cold pressed castor oil-hot water bottle or heating pad-white plastic (garbage bag)

Two or three one-foot squares of cotton flannel, wool, or towel

On top of the hot water bottle or heating pad, lay the plastic. Next soak the cloth with castor oil and lay this on top of the plastic. Lay plastic and/ or a towel underneath on the bedding. The entire

need 3 bowel movements a day. It is most important

-*Second procedure*: For the next 14 days, one tablespoon of slippery elm gruel five times a day. Either of these methods will coat, soothe and heal the lesions in the intestinal wall.

-*Third procedure*: For the next two days repeat the first procedure.

-*Fourth procedure:* Take copious (triple the stated dosages on the label) amounts of multi-strain Probiotic to re-establish the flora. Further aids would be to eat raw sauerkraut, Kim Chi, raw apple cider vinegar, Rejuvelac, or miso in large amounts; they rebuild the flora once the leaky gut is healed.

The pro-biotic need to be taken for about a week to rebuild the flora.

Note: do not feed the yeast during this procedure. Therefore, do not consume any sugar or alcohol in any form. This includes all dairy, grains, and fruit. Do eat vegetable, nuts, seeds and sprouted legume diet

Liver cleanse - gallbladder cleanse

Epsom salts 4 tablespoons in 3 cups of water +1/2 (half) cup (light olive oil is easier to get down), and for best results, ozonate it for 20 minutes. Add 2 drops hcl. +Fresh pink grapefruit 1 large or 2 small, enough to squeeze 2/3 cup juice. Hot wash twice first and dry each time. +Ornithine (amino acid) 4 to 8, to be sure you can sleep. Use Large plastic straw adds Black Walnut Tincture, strength 10 to 20 drops, to kill parasites coming from the liver.

-*Choose a day like Friday for the cleanse*, Take no medicines, vitamins or pills that you can do without; they could prevent success. Stop the parasite program and kidney herbs, too, the day before. Eat a no-fat breakfast and lunch such as cooked cereal, fruit, fruit juice, bread and preserves or honey (no butter or milk).

-*2:00 PM. Do not eat or drink after 2 o'clock*. If you break this rule you could feel quite ill later. Get your Epsom salts ready. Mix 4 tbs. In 3 cups water and pour this into a jar. This makes four servings, 3/4 (three fourths) cup each. Set the jar in the refrigerator to get ice cold (this is for convenience and taste only).

pack is then placed on the abdomen. The body can then be wrapped in a large bath towel. The pack should remain in place for at least an hour. It can be reused a few times, but it needs to be refrigerated. If very toxic, don't reuse it very much (use your intuition on this), as the pack draws the toxins out of the body. With each use, add a little more castor oil. Clean up with a little soda water. This treatment feels so nice.

CLAY CLEANSE-must take clay 1 hour before meals or 2 hours before medications (clay will absorb nutritious and make meds of no effect)

Important when taking clay: use distill and purify water only (do not use tap water) drink at least 1 gallon of liquid especially water

Never use metal container or spoons on clay- use wood or glass-clay can be stored in plastic when dry (once you add water only use glass container)

Clay pulls the heavy metal floating around in the body it does not affect metal implants-dose: children weighing 50lbs. Or less: 1/8 tsp. In 4 oz. Of water

Adult or children 50-100lbs. :1/2 tsp. In 4 oz. Water

Adults weighing 100-150 lbs. 1 tsp. In 8 oz. Water

Adults weighing 150-300 lbs. 2 tsp. In 16 oz. Water

Night before using clay: mix dose above let sit in the water overnight (makes clay more powerful)-let stand in glass for at least 8 hours

-----------------------------*Steps*-----------------------------

1st week: start : on a Sunday (each Sunday will be your start day,1st thing upon arising drink the top liquid only (leave the sludgy part - discard do not re-use)-do this for 7 days

2nd and 3rd week: mix night before but next day drink entire content of clay mixture

4th week: take no clay for 7 days

5th to 7th week: Repeat the process of week 2-3 do this for 3 weeks

8th week: take 7 days of rest

9th- 11th week: do same as week 5-7

You can substitute 3 cups water used in this recipe to dissolve Epsom salt with 3 cups freshly pressed grapefruit or orange or freshly pressed apple juice. That way you will not feel unpleasant taste of Magnesium Sulphate

-6:00 PM. Drink one serving 3/4 (three fourths cup) of the ice cold Epsom salts. If you did not prepare this ahead of time, mix 1 tbs. In 3/4 (three fourth) cup water now. You may add 1/8 (one eight) tsp. Vitamin C powder to improve the taste. You may also drink a few mouthfuls of water afterwards or rinse your mouth. Get the olive oil (ozonated, if possible) and grapefruit out to warm up.

-8:00 PM. Repeat by drinking another 3/4 (three fourths) cup of Epsom salts. You haven't eaten since two o'clock, but you won't feel hungry. Get your bedtime chores done. The timing is critical for success.

-9:45 PM. Pour 1/2 (half) cup (measured) olive oil into the pint jar. Add 2 drops hcl to sterilize. Wash grapefruit twice in hot water and dry; squeeze by

hand into the measuring cup. Remove pulp with fork. You should have at least 1/2 (half) cup, more (up to 3/4 (three fourths) cup) is best. You may use part lemonade. Add this to the olive oil. Also add Black Walnut Tincture. Close the jar tightly with the lid and shake hard until watery (only fresh grapefruit juice does this).

-10:00 PM. Drink the potion you have mixed. Take 4 <u>ornithine</u> capsules with the first sips to make sure you will sleep through the night. Take 8 if you already suffer from insomnia. Drinking through a large plastic straw helps it go down easier. You may use oil and vinegar salad dressing, or straight honey to chase it down between sips. Have these ready in a tablespoon on the kitchen counter. Take it all to your bedside if you want, but drink it standing up. Get it down within 5 minutes (fifteen minutes for very elderly or weak persons).

Lie down immediately. You might fail to get stones out if you don't. The sooner you lie down the more stones you will get out.

To detoxify the body using a clay bath: do not take more than 2 clay baths per week (it is pulling so much toxins -you will get weak)use 10-15 cups of clay per bath - do 1 bath the 1st week than the next week start doing 2 weekly

Do not stay longer than 30 minutes 1st week and max 45 minutes thereafter

(body will start to reabsorb the toxins)

Make sure the clay has no lumps and is well mixed in the tub (will clog pipe)

Do not use metal tubs - must be porcelain surface (plastic and fiberglass tubs are less recommended) 1/2 cups wormwood / black walnut- 1/2 cups bentonite clay *(omit if not getting colonic*

COFFEE ENEMA

*-function-*causes bile duct to dilate and portal vein draining poisons out causes the liver to produce more bile, opens the ducts and causes bile to flow.(dumping toxins)this relieves pain

If colonic not available / alternate with colonic in difficult cases

-fast on juices only for 10 days-during those 10 days take coffee enema -this causes preparation of coffee enema-add 3 rounded tbs. Of organic coffee to 1 qt. Of distilled water in a saucepan. Boil for 3 minutes uncovered; then cover, lower heat then simmer for an additional 15 minutes. Strain and cool. Add more water to make a full qt. (use at body temperature)

-note: - do enemas 1-2 daily and , when always during headaches, migraines , pain, nausea, constipation-after fasting for 10 days do recommended diet for post colonic

*-do clear water enema1st to clear the colon-*then place the coffee solution in an enema bag - hang bag at a 14- 24 inch height - instill solution while lying on right side, with both legs drawn close to the abdomen -(if the flow is too fast it will cause spasm, add chamomile to solution to stop spasm) -the fluid should be retained for 12-15 minutes have a stop watch on hand- the caffeine goes through the hemorrhoidal veins into the portal vein and into the liver-after 12-15 minutes, evacuate the enema into the toilet

Be ready for bed ahead of time. Don't clean up the kitchen. As soon as the drink is down walk to your bed and lie down flat on your back with your head up high on the pillow. Try to think about what is happening in the liver. Try to keep perfectly still for at least 20 minutes. You may feel a train of stones traveling along the bile ducts like marbles. There is no pain because the bile duct valves are open (thank you Epsom salts!). Go to sleep, you may fail to get stones out if you don't.

-Next morning. Upon awakening take your third dose of Epsom salts. If you have indigestion or nausea wait until it is gone before drinking the Epsom salts. You may go back to bed. Don't take this potion before 6:00 am.

-2 Hours Later. Take your fourth (the last) dose of Epsom salts. You may go back to bed again.

PART TEN
CLEANSE THERAPY

Only Use One Chosen Juice For The Three Days, and swish each mouthful thoroughly, (called chewing), so the saliva will mix with it; therefore our bodies can get all the nutrition and healing value from it.

Although if very hungry towards evening, you may take some celery. **When using apple juice, an apple or two is acceptable.**

Use only unsweetened juice containing no additives. Do not use frozen concentrate (it has been cooked). Use fresh grape juice, if possible.

Apples are one of the greatest herbs and blood purifiers known Fresh apple juice is best. Optional Carrot Juice Therapy /Apple juice/ Grape Juice Therapy

Citrus Juice Therapy:

four to six grapefruit, two to three lemons, and enough oranges to complete a total mixture of two quarts. Dilute using two quarts of distilled water, making one gallon of citrus juice mixture. Proceed as in the apple juice therapy.

Diabetic-dilute al juices with 50% distilled water, check blood sugar daily (add greens or barley green to the juice to slow digestion -consult physician-if sugar remains high, cut back the apple and carrots -use mostly greens for juices or water and barley green-drink the black poultice with water instead of juice -treat the liver beforehand with coffee enemas

Candida patients -use only granny smith apples, cranberries, lemon or lime for juice or eating and no other fruits for the 10 days

STEP FOUR: induce sweating TEA-Do not gives cold drinks. Instead, give those cups of hot diaphoretic tea, such as yarrow or another type. You will want to stay with only one type of tea. Have your patient drink as much as possible. This will keep the patient from a dry fever. You should give them a cup to drink about every 10 to 15 minutes.

Your patient may get lightheaded and feel like fainting. If so, place a cold towel or washcloth on their forehead. Leave the patient in the hot bath as long as possible; at least 45 minutes (may reduce for a small infant). You will know when to get a child out when perspiration starts to bead up on the face. At this point, give them 10 to 15 more minutes. *When your patient* is ready to leave the tub, you will need to lift him or her out, as they will be unable to support themselves. Fainting can occur when you pull the patient out of the bath. Keep a cayenne tincture on hand in case your patient goes into shock.

STEP FIVE: COLD SHEET THERAPY- when patient out of the bath, wrap the large double cotton sheet, dripping wet from being soaked in ice-cold water, around the standing patient. With just the head and the feet protruding, pin the sheet down the side. Help your patient into the prepared bed that has been covered with plastic and with a cotton sheet. Then place dry cotton sheet covers over the patient while they are still wrapped in the cold sheet. Add additional natural fiber blankets over the top of the sheet for warmth and to continue the sweating routine.

-use less carrots and more greens for juicing

-use fresh garlic (mix a finely chopped clove in a little water and drink)

Use cold sheet therapy

Use teas (liver cleanse, kidney, blood and bowel)

A.Diaphoretic Tea-Prepare a gallon of diaphoretic tea. This can be any good sweating herb, preferably yarrow. But it can also be blessed thistle, chamomile, pleurisy root, boneset, thyme, Hyssop, garden sage, catnip, spearmint, or any other good, diaphoretic herb.

For one gallon:1 cup of diaphoretic herb -1 gallon or 4 liters distilled water

Preparation: Pour boiling water over herbs, cover, allow to steep (not boil) in a warm place 30 minutes. Strain and sweeten with honey if desired. Keep warm until used.

Garlic Paste

To prepare a garlic paste for an adult, use 1 part garlic and 1 part petroleum jelly.

Reduce the amount of garlic for a child or small infant to 1 part garlic to 3 parts petroleum jelly. For an adult, you will want about 1 cup of paste.

Crush or finely grate peeled garlic cloves. Blend with an equal amount of petroleum jelly.

C. Hot Bath-Fill a hot tub of hot water. Add to the water, according to your tolerance, one or all of the following diaphoretic herbs, ginger being the mildest, then dry mustard, with cayenne as the most stimulant. Use *1 ounce* of each herb.

D. Bed with Plastic-Prepare a bed by placing a rubber or plastic sheet over the mattress, with a cotton sheet over it. Have several natural blankets on hand, such as wool or cotton.

E.Enema-4 tablespoons catnip, sage, or red raspberry cut or powdered herb

1 quart distilled water

STEP SIX: GARLIC PASTE-With your patient lying down in bed, thoroughly massage their feet from the ankles down with olive oil. Allow as much of this oil to be absorbed into the skin as possible, covering the soles, sides, and entire foot area. After you have massaged each foot, *prepare a strip of cotton that is wide enough to cover the bottom of the foot with ½ inch of the garlic paste.* When this is done, place the strip of cotton with the past on the sole of the foot, then take a roll of two-inch gauze and gently wrap the foot to secure the strip of garlic to the foot. With this in place, gently pull over the foot and gauze bandage a large white cotton wool sock to hold everything in place.

Do not allow the paste to get up on the sides or on top of the foot. Put it only on the sole. *Put the bandaged feet back* under the cold, wet sheet and pin the bottom of the sheet together so that the patient will be in a wet sack. You will want to use a large double sheet instead of small because it will allow your patient to roll or turn around without being too closely confined.

STEP SEVEN: SOUND Sleep-In most cases, your patient will sleep soundly all night in the cold sheet. You do not have to worry about them wanting to get up to urinate because of the large amount of tea they drank. While the body is in the cold, wet sheet, the subconscious mind will build an artificial fever to warm the body.

STEP EIGHT: SPONGE BATH-After your patient awakes out of the deep sleep, take them out of the bed and sponge them down thoroughly with a warm mixture of 1 part apple cider vinegar and 1 part distilled water 1 quart of solution, so use approximately 1 pint of each.

Put fresh clothing on the patient and fresh bedding on the bed.

Preparation: Bring distilled water to a boil and pour over cut herb. Steep for 30 minutes. Strain the herb and set in refrigerator until tea is cool. Pour tea into enema bucket or bag. Lubricate the end of the enema hose to be inserted into the rectum.

F. Garlic Injection (bulb syringe)

1 cup apple cider vinegar+1 cup distilled water+3 or more cloves of garlic

Preparation: Combine vinegar and water. Grate, squeeze through garlic press, or puree in blender 3 cloves of garlic until finely crushed. Blend in water and vinegar mixture. Put mixture into syringe and check flow. If flow is loose, add additional crushed garlic. Continue adding as much garlic as you can, making sure the mixture flows from syringe without clogging.

STEP ONE: CLEANSING COLD ENEMA

Give the patient an enema using catnip, sage, red raspberry or some other herb, but preferably catnip. You will want to administer this enema cold.

Important Note: <u>Do not use</u> enemas except in the case of emergencies.

STEP TWO: GARLIC INJECTION

In herbology an injection is never a needle; it is a syringe type application into an already existing orifice of the body, i.e. The rectum, ears, or nose. Insert the prepared injection into the rectum with a syringe. Use the full pint for an adult and less for a child. Have your patient retain the injection for as long as possible before voiding.

STEP THREE: HYDROTHERAPY

After the patient has expelled the garlic injection, help him or her into a hot bath prepared with diaphoretic herbs. Have the water as hot as your patient can possibly tolerate. Cayenne, dry mustard, and ginger will increase the perspiring of the patient by opening the pores wide.

STEP NINE: JUICE THERAPY-fresh fruit or vegetable juices -Fresh Vegetable and Fruit Juices or Wheat Grass drink in School of Natural Healing or bottled fresh grape juice, apple juice, etc., with no additives. Each mouthful of juice should be swished or chewed thoroughly to mix it with the saliva for good assimilation. In addition, chewing your juice will prevent an unpleasant sugar reaction if your patient is hypoglycemic or diabetic. *Do not mix* the patients juices. If a different juice is desired, wait at least one half hour before using a different one. During the day it is good for your patient to have as much distilled water as desired and some good herb teas. It is best to keep your patient on juice therapy for one to two days to allow thorough cleansing of the digestive organs before going into the Mucusless diet.

PART ELEVEN
JUICING

JUICING USE THESE COMBINATIONS	Use the numbers above for the following
1. Cabbage, carrots celery, kale 2. Beet tops, carrots, dandelion, garlic, black radish 3. Carrot, Swiss chard, celery, hawthorn berries 4. Carrot, celery, parsley, turnips, kale 5. Wheat grass, carrot, cabbage, celery, broccoli 6. Beets and tops, wheat grass, turnip greens, carrot, dandelion 7. Carrot, celery, parsley, cucumber, beets 8. Cranberry, apples, pears, grapes, papayas, pineapple (mix any three) 9. Watermelon, celery, parsley, cucumber 10. cranberrie, blueberry, orange, grapes, guava, mango, pineapple	Acne--------------------7 Allergy--------------7 Anemia-----------------1, 2, 6 Angina-----------------3 Arthritis------------3, 6, 8 Asthma----------------5 Blood cleaner---2, 6 Bladder---------------6, 8 Blood disorder—6 Cancer---------------1, 2, 5 Chronic illness-5 Colds-----------------4 Colitis---------------7 Colon disorder-1, 6, 8 Constipation------8 Dermatitis----------1 Digestion-----------4, 8 Diuretics-----------4 Edema----------------3, 4 Eye--------------------4 Gallbladder-----2, 8 Glands--------------2 Gout------------------7 Halitosis----------7 Hay fever---------7 Heart----------------2, 3, Hemorrhoids----3 Highpertention-3, 7 Infection----------10 Inflammation------4, 8 Intestines---------3, 5 Kidney---------------6 Liver-----------------2, 6(chronic) Osteoporosis----3, 6 Pancreatitis-----7 sinusitis------------7 Skin--------------------3, 7 Red blood cells –2 Ulcer-----------------1, 5 Urinary------------8 Varicose---(cabbage juice pulp to area) Weight loss------4, 7, 9

JUICING CLEANSE

Greens such as (collards, spinach, broccoli, parsley, wheat grass or dandelion greens- should make up no more than ¼ of the juice-the recipe should make 8-12 ounces-green superfood are optional

Breakfast

1 apple

1 beet

½ small lemon/ lime peeled

1 cup berries

3 oranges, peeled

1 scoop green superfood

1 grapefruit, peeled

½ small lemon/ lime peeled

1 scoop green superfood

1 scoop green superfood

4 carrots

root, a handful parsley

4 carrots, a handful spinach, collard greens or beet greens, 1 apple cut watermelon into sections juice enough to = 8-12 ounce-½ cantaloupe, 1 cup berries

4 handful of parsley

2 apples

4 carrots

1 scoop green superfood

2 apples

¼ inches sliver ginger root

½ small lemon/ lime

1 scoop superfood

Add water to make 8 oz.

1 cup strawberries, blueberries/ blackberries

1 pink grapefruit, peeled

1 scoop green superfood

Mid-morning snack

2 celery, 2 apples, 2 carrots-a handful of parsley, 4 carrots, 1 apple

2 carrots, 2 celery stalk, 1 apple, 1 beet

3 inch slice pineapple with skin, ¼ inch ginger

Lunch juices

1.2 celery stalk+4 carrots+ a handful parsley 1 garlic cloves

2.1 beet+ 2 carrots+2 celery stalk+ ½ sweet potatoes uncooked ¼-1/2 head of cabbage

3.handful collard greens, 2 carrots, 1 apple

4. A handful parsley, 1 tomatoes, 1 cucumber, 2 celery stalks 1 garlic cloves (optional)

5. 1 handful dandelion greens or 1 dandelion root,2 celery stalks, 4 carrots

6. 2 celery stalks, 2 carrots, 1 beets, ¼-1/2 head of cabbage

Evening juices

1.¼- ½ head cabbage, 2 celery stalk,½ cucumber

2. 4 medium potatoes,2 celery stalks, ½ cucumber,1 hand of alfalfa sprouts or broccoli sprouts, 1 garlic cloves (optional)

3. 2 carrots , 1 beet, ½ cucumber, 2 celery stalks

4. 4 carrots, a handful of collard greens, spinach or beet greens 1 garlic cloves, a handful parsley

5. 4 carrots, a handful dandelion greens or 1 dandelion root

Soups to use during fasting

-use dulse powder to spice them up

1. 2 garlic cloves, ½ cucumber, 2 celery stalk, a handful spinach

2. 4 carrots, 2 celery stalk, a handful parsley, 1 garlic cloves -¼-1/2 head cabbage, 2 celery stalk, 2 carrots, a handful parsley-1 cucumber, 2 tomatoes, a handful of parsley, 1 garlic clove

PART TWELVE
HYDROTHERAPY

Water temperature= in degree f.

  A. Hot water-------104-110

  B. Hot --------------100-104

  C. Neutral-----------94-97

  D. Warm-------------92-100

  E. Tepid-------------80-92

  F. Cool----------------70-80

  G. Cold----------------55-70

  H. Very cold---------32-55

Bath additives:

Epson salt=*(magnesium sulfate) a. Purpose -sore tired muscles* -it attracts carbon waste products and pull them out of the system

Procedure- put 1-3 lbs. Into bath water of 100-101f.-soak in tub for 30 minutes -(do not use soap)- it will bind with the salt making it ineffective-rest for 1 hour -keep hydrated

Mustard -*purpose*-to raise the body temperature and open the pores

-increase sweating and expel toxins-cold -congestion

Instructions -put 2 cups into hot bath (101-104f.)-soak for about 30 minutes -rest 1 hour after-keep well hydrated

Caution(get person out when complains of feeling hot)

Oatmeal: purpose-skin irritation (poison oak/ ivy, hives, rashes)

Ice massage:

Equipment- -ice in foam cup and freeze -towel

Procedure- -apply rub on area to area for several minutes (causes burning to aching then area will become numb)must keep moving the ice for 7-10 minutes -dry area-then exercise the area right after or massage

Caution-rheumatoid arthritis -stroke -when person is cold

Mustard plaster:(remove when person complains its hot)

Equipment:- 1 parts -mustard - 4 parts -flour (whole wheat)-mixing bowl

-water -rolling pin -saran wrap

*Procedure:-*same as charcoal poultice-leave on skin until slightly redness of skin begin-remove plaster and cover area to keep warm

*Caution:-*wash off if burning persist-if skin burn apply olive oil

Chest for congestion*mustard plaster*

Neutral bath :(94-97 f.)

Equipment-bath tub filled with water 94-97 degrees f. (depending on temperature of the room and the individual (may increase water temp. To 98-99 degrees f.)

-Bath thermometer -bath towel -air pillow or towels for head

Procedure: Keep in water for 30 minutes to as much as 5 hours-Remove from tub and dry-Rest in bed for at least 30 minutes

Procedure- blend 4 cups of oatmeal into powder-add to warm water-soak for 30 minutes to 1 hour

Charcoal: purpose- toxins removal-cold, flu-painful conditions

Procedure; -2 cup of activated charcoal in 1/2 qtr. Of water mix- add to bath water -keep person well hydrated during treatment

100-101f.-mix and soak for 20-30 minutes -rinse off and rest for 1 hour

Bath-hot foot bath:

Equipment needed: -bucket, thermometer, blanket, towel, bucket hot - water small container of cold water, cool water to drink

Procedure:-lay in bed , cover with sheet, put towel under hot water bucket

-put feet in 103 degree-f temp.-put cold towel on head (moving the congestion from the head) -keep adding more hot water(pick feet out of water before adding)

-give sips of water during treatment

-to finish treatment pick feet out of water and pour cold water on the feet

-have person lay and rest for 30 minutes after

Bath-local alternate bath:(contrast bath)

Equipment -2 tubs hot and cold 110 and 70 degrees-boiled water

-thermometer to check water -2 towel one for under the container other to dry area being treated-bucket of ice -pitcher to remove or add water or ice

Procedure:-put hand or effected area into the hot water for 3 minutes

-switch too cold for 30 seconds -switch back and forth (6-8 changes)-do 2-3x

During the day - adding hot or ice in basins to maintain temperature

-complete the treatment in cold for 30 seconds and dry area

Caution: -keep hot water temperature for diabetics and peripheral vascular disease at 104 degrees or below-caution in patients with tendency to hemorrhage

Caution:some cases of eczema -person with great heart weakness

Salt glow:

Equipment- -wet salt-2 cups of table salt moisture in a quart size container-pan of warm water-2 sheet -massage table or bed, standing or sitting-1 towel

Procedure: take warm shower - opt. Shampoo hair-wet each limb or area before applying salt friction turning the skin pink-Moisture skin with ice cold water -start with hand to ward chest -foot to hips -do chest- Do stomach-Do back-take a shower -Rest for 30 minutes

Shower-alternate cold and hot shower:

Procedure: -start with hot (100f. Raising) water for 1 minute switch too cold for 30 sec. Repeat this alternating hot and cold (make 3 complete cycle ending with hot- cold)-last heat cycle gradually lower the temperature to neutral (94-97 f.) For 1 1/2 minutes -last cold cycle do for 15 seconds

-during the cold have person rub skin with hands-Have person rest for 30-60minutes

Cautions:do not use with appendicitis (or an acute condition)- Acute nervous

Irritability or excitability-poor circulation (may faint).severe cardiovascular disease

Skin brushing:(can be done daily)*do not use on skin lesions or rashes*

Purpose: a. Exfoliating skin- b. Dry or inactive skin c.to improve overall health

D. All chronic disease (diabetes, hypertension, circulatory insufficiency, cardiac insufficiency, cancer)

Equipment: a. Natural bristle brush -b. Olive oil for dry skin

Procedure: more vigorous the brushing=more effective

A. Lay in bed -b. Start with hands to arm to shoulder (brush skin) -c. Feet to legs to hips d. Do chest to abdomen to back to buttocks

E. Finish with neutral bath and oil the skin with olive if dry

Bath Cold local bath

*Equipment:-*container large enough to cover area being treated(60 degree water)-thermometer-pitcher to add ice or cold water -ice -2 towels procedure -place feet in area for 30 minutes (causing vasoconstriction-relieving pain)-remove and dry area

Caution-person with diabetes, and vascular disease-care should be taken to prevent chilling

Bath-hot tub bath (boost immune system) 100-104 degrees

Equipment; bath thermometer-basin of ice water-2 wash cloth for compresses

-2-3 bath towels-folded bath towels for pillow- If prolonged : ice bag and water to Drink -Thermometer for checking body temperature

*Procedure:(*room warm and free from draft)-keep for a minimum of 10 minutes to 20 minutes -fill tub 2/3 full(if room is cold is cold cover exposed body part with a towel) put cool compress on head (keep changing it) check body oral temperature and pulse on carotid artery -check every 3-5 minutes (keep heart rate less than 115 beats per minutes-keep body temperature less than 102 degree (give glass of water)-communicate with person for (dizzy, weakness) -at termination of treatment apply cool water to spine while kneeling in tub then cool shower -assist person may faint- Dry off (drink a glass of water) - cover and rest for 30 minutes

Caution**: *heart rate rises over 115 beats per minutes (put ice bag over heart)*

Don't do for heart patients and diabetes aged or feeble, high blood pressure,

Circulatory problems-Never leave person unattended

-persons on pharmaceutical drugs should proceed with cautions

-infants and small children should be treated same as the feeble

Charcoal poultice:

*Equipment:-*1/4 cups activated charcoal- 1/4 cups psyllium seed husk (or flax seed meal)-1cups water -saran wrap-rolling pin (opt.)

Steam inhalation:

Equipment; tea kettle to boil water-Towel or (newspaper cone) for concentrating vapor for inhalation-Hot plate-eucalyptus oil, pine oil. For medicating airway

Procedure: plug in steamer -Put a few medicated oil in their For 10 minutes at a time with 1 hour break in between because it heats the brain

Caution: Avoid burns, children and elderly do for a shorter duration. Chronic

Respiratory disease or chronic heart disease may get shortness of breath

Sun bath:starts for 5 minutes working up daily for up to 20 minutes

Caution: -heat stroke -lupus (not the face and short exposure time)

Russian steam bath:

Equipment:-tea kettle and hot plate / or plug in tea kettle-plastic or wooden chair -.plastic sheeting or shower curtain-hot foot bath(5 gallon bucket or container 1/2 full)with 103 f. Water to start- then warm up to 106-110f. Depending on tolerance to heat-2 towels-drinking water and straw

-cold compress (small container with cold water and medium- sized towels)

*Procedure:-*place steam kettle under chair covered with sheet have spout pointing back away from person -put plastic on floor and towel under foot bath-chest temperature for base line -sit person on chair -drape a towel over persons shoulder to protect from plastic

-drape plastic over person, footbath and steam kettle

-keep head cool-wrap cold compress around neck, and head-check body temperature often

-offer drink of water (at least 2-3 glasses during treatment)-keep body temperature about 102 degrees -keep foot temp around 106-110 degree range-keep in treatment for 7 minutes - for stimulation only for disease keep in for 15minutes-to finish- cool shower- cover with sheet and lay for 30-60 minutes

-something to secure charcoal (ea. Ace wrap)-mixing bowl

*Procedure:-*mix charcoal + psyllium seed or flax seed -add water till gel

-put mixture on saran wrap and roll out till 1/4 inch thickness-let set 3-5 minutes-take off side of saran and apply to area and use bandage to hold poultice in place -if using for pain leave on overnight or several hours during the day -for spider or snake bites change it every 15-20 minutes

-can refrigerate indefinitely

Fomentations:(moist heat to body part)

Procedure: -dry towel to area -constant communication to person for comfort-put heating pad on tower and cover for 3-5 minutes -remove and do cold friction rub to area cold towel (wet)- vigorously rub area for 30 seconds and dry area and reapply heat

Fomentation for chest congestion: do exchange 3-5x

Procedure: -put plastic on bed (for protection) -lay sheet on bed with towel across top and foot where foot basin will be

-place hot moist pad on bed at chest area(roll several in plastic put in microwave ready for use) heat for 5 minutes in microwave all at once

-open one hot fomentation pad on dry towel and cover

-put towel along spine and place pad on top-lay patient down

-put dry towel on chest-put fomentation on chest and cover to hold heat in

-cover with a blanket and sheet and tuck under hot foot bath

-keep cool compress to head and neck

-if complain of too hot to an area put another towel to skin of that area

-after 5 minutes make an exchange of chest fomentation after (doing a 30 second vigorous chest cold friction) and dry the chest

Special note: Hot herbal tea will assist in sweating-rubbing the body during

Treatment will help the body to sweat and assist in exfoliation of skin

also will relieve feelings of nausea, weakness, and dizziness

Treatment needs to be given on an empty stomach 3 hours after a meal

Caution: *If head and neck are not kept cool- (headache, fatigue and depression will result)*

*Diabete*s-hot foot bath 103f. Or less +short duration

Hypertension- if heart beat gets 120 per minute or more place ice bag over heart (short treatment-working up to a long treatment)

Multiple sclerosis- hot treatment are very debilitating time limit usually 20 minutes

Wet sheet pack

(wet sheet pack(cooling stage)-tonic stage) (a little less than stimulating) procedure: -put plastic on bed -put a wool blanket on the bed (use 2blankets one on top of the other) if not wool use more than 2 blankets...-open a large sheet and fold both sides towards the middle until small enough than fold the other direction until small enough to fit in basin

-wet sheet(cold water-60-70 degrees)wrung sheet out and unfold in the bed and put person in the center - raise arm and roll sheet on body taking under 1 leg put hands down fold the other side over arms and entire body (tuck in)

-cover with the 2 blankets 1 at a time tucking it in-put towel around neck to keep heat in -put cold compress on head

Equipment: hot foot bath material-cold compress material-bucket of cold water 55-70f.

-2 large wool blankets(with others as many as needed)-1 large sheet-1 bath towel-plastic sheeting -if doing treatment on a bed

-finish with cold mitten friction + pour cool water to feet or cool shower

Notes: when used for lung congestion or congestion of other organs make 5 exchanges instead of 3 (use a cold compress to head and a hot foot bath)

-heart rate rise above 120 beat per minute (put ice bag to heart)

-if this treatment used for nervous states such as (insomnia) and nervous tensions use warm temperature instead of hot for 6-10 minutes (omit cold rub)-to relieve spasm do 3 exchanges

-for chronic inflammatory condition 5-10minutes 3 rotations every 2-3 hours

Heating compress:

Procedure: a. Wring cold sleeveless t- shirt in water and put it on

B. Wrap securely with no air pocket with wool pin and secure (cover wet shirt securely) c. Put a throat compress wet a flannel material and wrap with wool d. Put a sweatshirt over (leave overnight)

Caution:-do not use if weak, emaciated- will worsen conditionbecause body has no means of nutrient when vessels dilate as the compress warms the superficial vessels dilates, bringing blood to the surface-(relieving deeper congestion)

Special notes: -have patient void before treatment
-never leave person alone

-may use a hot water bottle at the feet to help heat person

Caution:-skin eruption, diabetics, severe colds or
-feeble- do not use (person cannot warm sheet)

INDEX